International Perspectives and Experiences Enhancing Access to Healthcare

Edited by Ronald J. Ozminkowski

Published in London, United Kingdom

International Perspectives and Experiences Enhancing Access to Healthcare
http://dx.doi.org/10.5772/intechopen.1003558
Edited by Ronald J. Ozminkowski

Contributors
Alejandro Jose Duarte Cuellar, Brandon Young, Charles Tobin-West, Chonin Cheang, Deneke Wolde, Feyissa Regassa Senbato, Gudeta D. Fufaa, Humberto Alcides Urbina Vasquez, Ifeyinwa Onwelumadu, Japheth David, Kasu T. Bifa, Luis Alberto Camputaro, Pedro Jofre Lora, Phil Salinger, Ronald J. Ozminkowski, Sandip Gupta, Suning Zhao, Tesfaye G. Bikila, Theresa Abah, Weiyee Lee, Wendy M. Smith, Wengtong Chan, Yejide Olukemi Oseni

First published in London, United Kingdom, 2025 by IntechOpen
IntechOpen is the global imprint of INTECHOPEN LIMITED, registered in England and Wales, registration number: 11086078, 167-169 Great Portland Street, London, W1W 5PF, United Kingdom

For EU product safety concerns: IN TECH d.o.o., Prolaz Marije Krucifikse Kozulić 3, 51000 Rijeka, Croatia, info@intechopen.com or visit our website at intechopen.com.

British Library Cataloguing-in-Publication Data
A catalogue record for this book is available from the British Library

International Perspectives and Experiences Enhancing Access to Healthcare
Edited by Ronald J. Ozminkowski
p. cm.

This title is part of the Public Health Book Series, Volume 1
Series Editor: José Antonio Mirón Canelo

Print ISBN 978-0-85014-748-3
Online ISBN 978-0-85014-747-6
eBook (PDF) ISBN 978-0-85014-749-0
ISSN 3049-8872

IntechOpen Book Series
Public Health
Volume 1

Aims and Scope of the Series

Public health is what we as a society do collectively to contribute to and ensure the health and social conditions for the enjoyment of health as a resource for life. It can also be defined as science and research that promotes health, prevents disease, and improves populations' well-being and quality of life. Its objective is to know the risk factors that determine and condition the populations' health levels at present. At the end of the 20th century and the beginning of the 21st century, it is unjustifiable and regrettable that morbimortality according to age plays a leading role when the causes are mostly well known and therefore preventable, such as obesity, AIDS, cirrhosis, diabetes mellitus, addictions and cancer associated with the consumption of tobacco and alcohol, etc. In short, public health is science based on epidemiology and biostatistics, and currently, new technologies and artificial intelligence must be incorporated to identify patterns and trends in what we do collectively as a society to ensure living conditions and prevent risk factors that affect individual and population health. For all these reasons, it is essential to scientifically investigate and act on the determinants that impede the well-being and quality of life related to the health of people, patients, and populations in general, given that to control the determinants of diseases, it is important to control the environment and genetics. Consequently, the current fight for public health must prioritize the control of the environment, such as atmospheric and biological pollution and environmental and social biodiversity, promoting the sensitivity and training of society and its individuals by empowering them to make free and appropriate decisions about these aspects to lead healthy lifestyles based on motivation and responsibility in the face of the challenges they cope with from an individual point of view, such as dealing with the addictions that exist in today's complex world. Public health also requires an ethical vision and incorporates strategies to reduce social inequality.

Meet the Series Editor

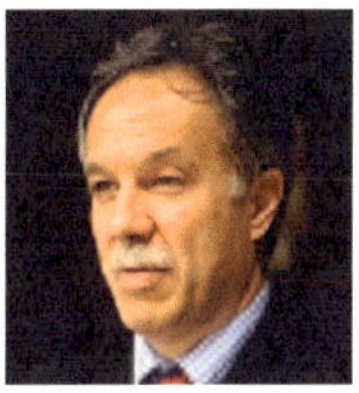

José Antonio Mirón Canelo is a physician, doctor, and professor of Preventive Medicine and Public Health at the Faculty of Medicine and Dentistry of the University of Salamanca with over 30 years of experience. He is the director of the USAL's Expert Degree in Health Management, currently in its 13th edition. Prof. Mirón Canelo directs a research group at the Research Institute of Biomedical Sciences (IBSAL) of the University of Salamanca focused on addressing the challenges and care needs of vulnerable people and patients such as the elderly with multiple pathologies and people with disabilities and dependence. As a teacher, he has been recognized for excellence in teaching three times in a period of five years.

Meet the Volume Editor

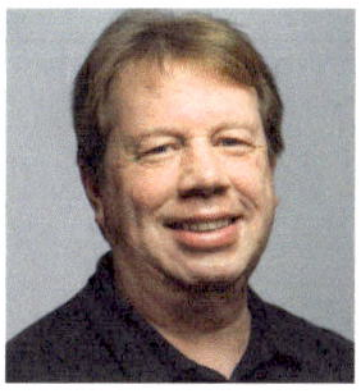

Ronald J. Ozminkowski, Ph.D., is an internationally recognized executive leader, consultant, writer, and chief scientist whose research has been viewed by people in more than 100 countries. He is a strategic thought leader, exemplified by his more than 300 peer-reviewed and other professional publications and conference presentations. His publications report investigations of access to care, social determinants of health and wellbeing, and evaluations of the impact of government and private sector clinical, pharmaceutical, and social programs designed to improve health and healthcare. His research collaborators and clients have included experts in the White House, federal and state agencies, life sciences companies, employers and insurers, pharmaceutical companies, industry groups, and health systems.

Contents

Preface

Ever since humanity evolved on this planet, we've individually and collectively faced many challenges in accessing the health care we need. One might think we would have resolved these issues for everyone by now, but here we are still trying, sometimes succeeding but often falling short. This book explores these challenges and potential solutions. Section 1, "Perspectives on Access, Quality, and Cost" includes three chapters. Section 2, "International Experiences", consists of five chapters discussing what has worked well and could likely work well at a larger scale if adopted in more places.

To frame the discussion, we begin by revisiting the key components of access to healthcare defined and tested decades ago by Roy Penchansky and J William Thomas [1]. Their model, known as the "Five-A's of Access," includes affordability, availability, accessibility, acceptability, and accommodation. This framework focuses on the needs of patients, providers, and payers.

The Five-A's have inspired researchers and practitioners for decades. My most recent examples come from presentations at the John R. Griffith Leadership Center for Health Management and Policy in Ann Arbor, Michigan. Discussions at the Center's annual event in October 2024 illustrated how the ability to pay for and receive necessary, culturally acceptable, convenient, and high-quality care has guided thinking across the United States, particularly about how to set up equitable healthcare services that also address challenges associated with social determinants of health.

Access problems, as well as the Five-A's, are global challenges. Section 1 of this book includes perspectives from Africa, Asia, and Central America, offering actionable strategies to improve access worldwide.

In Chapter 1, Feyissa Regassa Senbato, Deneke Wolde, Kasu T. Bifa and Tesfaye Gudissa review the factors that either facilitate or hinder access to health care. They propose policies to improve access in low- and middle-income countries and communities, such as expanding insurance coverage, using sliding-scale fees, introducing telemedicine options, building new facilities, and using mobile clinics to improve accessibility, acceptability, and accommodation barriers. The authors also discuss workforce policies to improve access and the utility of involving community health members in access-enabling interventions.

In Chapter 2, my coauthors and I build upon this foundation by describing how a new Health Equity and Affordability Tool (HEAT) and its Export Report can help employers tailor benefit plans and programs so insured members can manage the chronic conditions they have in better ways. The chapter also shows how coverage offerings can improve satisfaction with the health plans employees choose, enhance quality of care, and find acceptable and accommodating lower-cost providers. While HEAT has been developed for employers in the United States, its concepts apply internationally. It may be tailored for use in countries with similar input data.

In Chapter 3, Luis Alberto Camputaro, Humberto Alcides Urbina Vásquez, and Alejandro Jose Duarte Cuellar describe a growing system of air- and sea-based training programs to improve emergency response in El Salvador. Something like this may be helpful in many other countries around the globe. Leaders should establish international partnerships with treatment facilities within and between several neighbouring countries. Political or geographical trade barriers may complicate expanding the author's ideas, but so what? Progress is always painful in some ways, and humans can be quite innovative when facing these challenges.

Section 2 begins with Chapter 4, by Yejide Olukemi Oseni. The chapter presents quantitative and qualitative research describing why community pharmacists (CPs) should be authorized to provide COVID-19 vaccinations in Nigeria. Pairing descriptions of quantitative and qualitative approaches lends validity and context to the author's results. The randomization scheme for her qualitative survey and its high response rate also support her study's validity. The author also points out several factors that will bode well for the success of using CPs in the future. She notes that success in this endeavor will require formal policy changes, such as recognizing CPs as healthcare providers. Additional training so more CPs can be authorized to provide vaccinations is required, and much more funding is needed to expand access to vaccinations and deal with important idiosyncrasies, such as the ability to cold-store COVID-19 and/or other vaccines throughout Nigeria. Oseni stresses the need for collaboration across government agencies, professional organizations and non-government organizations to facilitate vaccination processes and lead to better outcomes. Her recommendations may also apply to many other countries within and beyond Africa.

In Chapter 5, Gudeta Fufaa provides a well-written primer on preventive services. He describes interventions designed to improve access to screening for several health conditions and the impact of those interventions. He briefly reviews successes and failures, focusing on access issues, and notes lessons important for public policy, insurers, employers, and future research on access. Fufaa also advises readers to consider screening policies related to environmental or employment-related factors, poverty, and other social determinants of health.

Moving on to Chapter 6, Japheth David and Charles Tobin-West offer a thoughtful and well-organized description of the challenges in obtaining adequate access to reproductive services in five African countries. The logical structure and content of their chapter are quite informative and will be useful for researchers and policymakers on other continents as well. Their focus on maternal mortality rates and ratios helps readers understand challenges and goals and provides context for considering many pragmatic solutions suggested by the authors. Their analysis highlights shared barriers, such as limited family planning services, low health literacy, and insufficient funding for women's health programs. The authors propose inclusive strategies to reduce maternal mortality and improve reproductive care, offering lessons for other regions worldwide.

In Chapter 7, Theresa Abah and Ifeyinwa Onwelumadu make a strong case to enhance access by integrating primary care and hospital care to serve people better. The authors illustrate the need to integrate medical care with interventions to avoid access barriers associated with social determinants of health. They also explore the growing importance of mental health integration and power imbalances within healthcare systems, offering a fresh perspective on addressing inequities.

Finally, Chapter 8 by Chonin Cheang, Wengtong Chan, and Sunning Zhao presents a case study of the strategic planning history of access to healthcare in Macau. They describe how public/private partnerships have been leveraged to improve the recruiting and retention of healthcare providers. They describe how integrations with the Guangdong Hong Kong Greater Bay Area (GBA) increased access to care and technology in Macau. Integrating Traditional Chinese Medicine with modern healthcare services offers a promising model for other regions to explore.

I hope this book inspires and motivates readers to view access barriers as surmountable challenges. I want to thank all the contributing authors as well as the staff at IntechOpen, especially Publishing Process Manager Dominik Samardzija and Senior Commissioning Editor Iva Simcic Mance. Thank you, dear readers, for engaging with this volume. I wish you success in your efforts to improve health and health care across our diverse planet.

Ronald J. Ozminkowski, PhD
Commercial Analytics,
Aon plc,
Chicago, USA

Reference

[1] Penchansky R, Thomas JW. The concept of access: Definition and relationship to consumer satisfaction. Medical Care. Feb 1981;**19**(2):127-140. DOI: 10.1097/00005650-198102000-00001. PMID: 7206846

Section 1

Perspectives on Access, Quality, and Cost

Chapter 1

Perspective Chapter: Strategies for Enhancing Healthcare Access

Feyissa Regassa Senbato, Deneke Wolde, Kasu T. Bifa and Tesfaye G. Bikila

Abstract

Strategies for enhancing healthcare access involve a multifaceted approach aimed at improving the availability, affordability, and quality of healthcare services for all individuals. These strategies may include initiatives to reduce financial barriers such as subsidies or insurance coverage, improve infrastructure and healthcare facilities in underserved areas, implement telemedicine and mobile health technologies to reach remote populations, foster community engagement and education to promote health literacy, and advocate for policy changes to address systemic inequalities. The aim of enhancing healthcare access is to overcome barriers such as geographic distance, financial constraints, lack of healthcare infrastructure, and limited availability of healthcare providers. Ultimately, the goal is to ensure that everyone can access essential healthcare services when needed, regardless of their socioeconomic status, geographical location, or other factors that may limit access. By implementing these strategies, healthcare access can be expanded, leading to improved health outcomes and greater equity in healthcare delivery.

Keywords: strategies, enhancing, healthcare, access, healthcare access

1. Introduction

Healthcare access refers to the ability of individuals to obtain necessary health services in a timely, convenient, and affordable manner. This concept encompasses not only the availability of services but also factors such as the quality, affordability, and acceptability of care provided to diverse populations [1]. Equitable healthcare access ensures that all individuals, regardless of their socioeconomic status, geographic location, or cultural background, can access the healthcare they need to achieve optimal health outcomes [2].

1.1 Importance of equitable access to healthcare

Equitable access to healthcare is crucial for maintaining public health, improving individual well-being, and reducing health disparities. Ensuring that healthcare is accessible to all promotes early detection and treatment of diseases, which can prevent complications and reduce overall healthcare costs [3]. Equitable access is also essential for fostering social justice and enhancing the overall quality of life within communities [4]. When healthcare access is equitable, it empowers populations to participate fully in society and contributes to the overall economic productivity of a nation [5].

Despite the critical importance of equitable access, numerous barriers persist that prevent many individuals from receiving appropriate care. Geographical barriers, such as living in rural or remote areas, can limit access to healthcare facilities and providers [6]. Financial barriers, including high out-of-pocket (OOP) costs and a lack of insurance coverage, pose significant challenges, particularly for low-income individuals and families [3]. Cultural barriers, such as language differences, mistrust of healthcare providers, and traditional health beliefs, can also hinder access to services, particularly for minority and immigrant populations [7]. Moreover, systemic factors, such as fragmented healthcare systems and inadequate infrastructure, further exacerbate these challenges; making it difficult for vulnerable populations to obtain the care they need [8].

Addressing these barriers requires a comprehensive approach that incorporates policy changes, technological innovations, community engagement, and targeted interventions designed to meet the needs of diverse populations. By understanding and tackling these obstacles, we can move toward a more inclusive and effective healthcare system that serves everyone.

2. Policy and regulatory strategies for enhancing healthcare access

Policy and regulatory strategies play a pivotal role in enhancing healthcare access by addressing systemic barriers and promoting equitable access to health services. Effective policies can reduce financial burdens, improve the availability of services, and ensure that healthcare is accessible to all segments of the population [3]. Key strategies include the expansion of health insurance coverage, implementation of government policies that promote healthcare access, and health reforms aimed at improving the delivery of care.

2.1 Expansion of health insurance coverage

Expanding health insurance coverage is one of the most effective ways to improve healthcare access, especially for low-income individuals and vulnerable populations. Health insurance provides financial protection, reduces out-of-pocket expenses, and increases the likelihood of individuals seeking timely medical care [9]. Policies such as Medicaid expansion in the United States have demonstrated significant improvements in access to healthcare services, particularly among previously uninsured groups [10].

By increasing the number of insured individuals, health systems can better manage healthcare costs and ensure that preventive and curative services are available to those who need them most [11].

2.2 Government policies promoting healthcare access

Government policies that promote healthcare access are critical in addressing the geographical, financial, and social barriers that hinder individuals from receiving necessary care. Policies that invest in healthcare infrastructure, such as building new facilities in underserved areas and improving transportation to healthcare services, can greatly enhance access, especially in rural and remote regions [12]. Additionally, policies that provide subsidies or reduce the cost of essential medications help alleviate the financial burden on patients, making healthcare more affordable and accessible [13]. Governments also play a crucial role in regulating healthcare providers to ensure that services are not only available but also meet quality standards that ensure patient safety and satisfaction.

2.3 Role of health reforms in improving access

Health reforms are designed to address systemic inefficiencies in healthcare delivery and to create a more inclusive and responsive health system. Reforms such as the Affordable Care Act (ACA) in the United States have shown how policy changes can significantly reduce the number of uninsured individuals and improve access to primary and preventive care [14]. Health reforms often include provisions for expanding coverage, improving healthcare quality, and increasing accountability among healthcare providers, all of which contribute to enhanced access [15]. Furthermore, reforms that prioritize patient-centered care models, such as value-based care, shift the focus from volume to quality, ensuring that patients receive appropriate, timely, and cost-effective care [16].

Through the implementation of targeted policy and regulatory strategies, governments can dismantle the barriers that prevent individuals and communities from accessing healthcare. By expanding insurance coverage, promoting supportive policies, and enacting meaningful reforms, healthcare systems can move closer to achieving universal access and improved health outcomes for all.

3. Improving healthcare infrastructure

Improving healthcare infrastructure is crucial for enhancing access to healthcare, particularly in underserved and remote areas. The following strategies address key approaches for overcoming the barriers to healthcare access.

3.1 Building healthcare facilities in underserved areas

One of the most direct ways to enhance healthcare access is by building healthcare facilities in underserved regions. In many low- and middle-income countries (LMICs), there is a pronounced disparity in the distribution of healthcare services, with rural and remote areas often lacking essential healthcare infrastructure [17]. Expanding infrastructure in these regions ensures that marginalized populations can access basic healthcare services, reducing the need for long-distance travel to urban centers for treatment. Building facilities with a focus on sustainability and adapting to local needs is also essential in ensuring long-term success [18].

3.2 Telemedicine and digital health platforms

Telemedicine and digital health platforms have emerged as innovative solutions to bridge the healthcare access gap, particularly in areas where building new infrastructure may not be feasible in the short term.

Telemedicine allows healthcare providers to consult with patients remotely, using digital platforms, and can be especially valuable in rural areas where specialist care is limited [19]. These platforms also facilitate the use of electronic health records, remote monitoring, and online consultations, which reduce travel time and costs for patients while expanding access to specialized care [20].

3.3 Mobile clinics and community outreach programs

Mobile clinics and community outreach programs provide flexible and adaptable healthcare services, particularly to populations that are geographically isolated or unable to access permanent healthcare facilities. These initiatives deliver essential services such as vaccinations, maternal health check-ups, and chronic disease management directly to the community [21, 22]. Mobile health units can also be rapidly deployed in response to health emergencies or outbreaks, offering critical care to vulnerable populations in real time. By utilizing community health workers (CHWs) and engaging local leaders, these programs help build trust and awareness, ensuring better uptake of health services in hard-to-reach areas [23].

4. Financial strategies to reduce cost barriers

One of the major challenges to healthcare access, particularly in LMICs, is the financial burden on patients. High out-of-pocket costs, lack of financial resources, and the absence of health insurance limit access to essential healthcare services [24]. To address these challenges, a range of financial strategies can be employed to make healthcare more affordable for all.

4.1 Subsidies and financial aid programs

Subsidies and financial aid programs are essential tools to alleviate the economic burden on individuals who cannot afford healthcare. These programs can be designed by governments, non-governmental organizations (NGOs), or healthcare institutions to cover part or all of the healthcare costs for low-income populations. For example, in many LMICs, governments provide healthcare subsidies for essential services such as maternal and child health or infectious disease treatment [25]. These programs often focus on key services, ensuring that even the poorest populations can access critical care without falling into financial hardship [26].

4.2 Sliding fee scales and payment plans

Sliding fee scales and flexible payment plans offer an alternative solution for reducing the financial barriers to healthcare.

Sliding fee scales adjust the cost of services based on a patient's income, ensuring that healthcare remains affordable regardless of economic status. This approach is widely used in community health centers and clinics, particularly in rural or underserved areas, to make care accessible to all income levels [27]. Payment plans, on the other hand, allow patients to spread the cost of their medical expenses over time, making it easier for individuals with limited financial means to afford necessary treatments without facing immediate financial strain [3].

4.3 Reducing out-of-pocket expenses for patients

Out-of-pocket (OOP) expenses remain one of the largest barriers to healthcare access, particularly in countries where health insurance coverage is limited or unavailable. To reduce these costs, governments and healthcare providers can implement policies that cap or reduce the expenses patients must pay for medical services and prescription drugs [28]. Additionally, expanding insurance coverage to include a broader range of services can significantly reduce OOP costs. Ensuring that essential health services such as preventive care, chronic disease management, and emergency care are covered by insurance or provided free of charge is crucial for reducing financial strain on patients [29]. By reducing these costs, healthcare systems can improve accessibility, prevent delays in seeking care, and mitigate the financial consequences of health crises for families.

5. Workforce development and distribution

A well-distributed and adequately trained healthcare workforce is critical to improving healthcare access, particularly in underserved and rural areas where shortages of health professionals are common. Effective workforce strategies can help bridge this gap and ensure that all populations receive the care they need.

5.1 Training and deploying healthcare professionals in rural and underserved areas

One of the most effective strategies for addressing healthcare access disparities is to train and deploy healthcare professionals in rural and underserved regions. Training programs should emphasize the specific healthcare needs of these communities, such as prevention and control of infectious diseases, maternal and child health, and basic primary care. Targeted recruitment from rural areas can also help ensure that professionals return to serve their communities, fostering trust and continuity of care [30].

Countries that have invested in rural health training programs have seen improvements in the distribution of healthcare workers and, consequently, in healthcare outcomes [31].

5.2 Task-shifting and community health worker programs

Task-shifting, the delegation of certain healthcare duties of less specialized health workers, is another strategy to address workforce shortages in underserved areas. Community health workers (CHWs) play a key role in this model, providing essential care and health education at the community level. CHWs, often trained in the basics of primary healthcare, maternal and child health, and chronic disease management, can extend healthcare services to areas where fully trained doctors and nurses may be scarce [32]. This approach has been successfully implemented in LMICs, where CHW programs have significantly improved healthcare delivery and patient outcomes in rural and isolated communities [33].

5.3 Incentives for healthcare providers in underserved regions

Providing financial and nonfinancial incentives for healthcare workers to practice in underserved regions is essential for ensuring a stable and committed workforce. Incentives such as salary bonuses, housing allowances, and opportunities for career advancement can motivate professionals to work in rural or hard-to-reach areas [34].

In addition to monetary incentives, offering continuous professional development opportunities, mentorship, and support for healthcare workers in these regions can enhance job satisfaction and retention [35]. Some countries have also implemented student loan repayment programs or scholarships for health professionals willing to serve in underserved areas for a set number of years, further improving the distribution of healthcare workers.

6. Role of community engagement and advocacy

Community engagement and advocacy play a vital role in enhancing healthcare access, particularly for marginalized populations. By involving communities in healthcare planning and decision-making, promoting healthcare rights, and fostering grassroots movements, healthcare systems can become more responsive to the needs of their populations.

6.1 Involving communities in healthcare planning and decision-making

Involving communities in healthcare planning and decision-making ensures that healthcare policies and programs reflect the specific needs and challenges faced by those they serve. Engaging local communities allows healthcare providers to better understand cultural, social, and economic factors that affect health outcomes. This participatory approach leads to the development of more effective, culturally sensitive, and sustainable health interventions [36]. Evidence shows that when communities are empowered to contribute to healthcare decisions, there is an improvement in health outcomes, trust in the health system, and overall patient satisfaction [37–39]. Community health boards, local health councils, and citizen advisory panels are examples of mechanisms through which communities can be actively involved in healthcare planning.

6.2 Advocacy for healthcare rights and access

Advocacy is crucial for ensuring that everyone has access to healthcare, regardless of their socioeconomic status, geographic location, or cultural background. Advocacy efforts aim to highlight healthcare disparities and push for policies that improve access to healthcare services, particularly for underserved populations [40]. Health advocacy organizations, civil society groups, and community leaders work together to ensure that healthcare remains a priority in public policy and that all individuals have access to affordable and quality care. Advocating for healthcare rights not only raises awareness about existing barriers but also strengthens the voices of vulnerable populations in policy-making [41].

6.3 Grassroots movements and community-led health initiatives

Grassroots movements and community-led health initiatives have proven effective in addressing specific health challenges at the local level. These initiatives are often initiated by local leaders or community members who are directly affected by health issues. Grassroots efforts are key in mobilizing communities to address pressing health concerns, such as maternal and child health, infectious diseases, and environmental health hazards [42].

Community-led health programs, including vaccination drives, sanitation projects, and health education campaigns, are instrumental in improving health outcomes, particularly in resource-poor settings [43].

These initiatives often leverage local resources and knowledge, leading to more sustainable health interventions.

7. Monitoring and evaluation of healthcare access strategies

Effective monitoring and evaluation (M&E) are crucial components for ensuring the success of healthcare access strategies. These processes enable stakeholders to measure the impact of interventions, utilize data to inform healthcare initiatives, and continuously improve access strategies, leading to more equitable and effective healthcare systems.

7.1 Measuring the impact of healthcare access interventions

To understand the effectiveness of healthcare access interventions, it is essential to measure their impact on the target population. This involves tracking key indicators, such as changes in service utilization, patient outcomes, and population health metrics. Evaluation frameworks like the RE-AIM model (Reach, Effectiveness, Adoption, Implementation, and Maintenance) are commonly used to assess the effectiveness of healthcare access initiatives [44]. In addition, baseline data collection, periodic surveys, and outcome evaluations help determine whether interventions are achieving their goals, such as improving access in underserved areas or reducing disparities in healthcare provision [45]. Regular impact assessments enable program managers and policymakers to adjust strategies based on real-world outcomes.

7.2 Using data to improve healthcare access initiatives

Data is an invaluable tool in shaping healthcare access strategies. By systematically collecting and analyzing health data, organizations can identify gaps in service delivery, population groups with unmet healthcare needs, and barriers to care. For example, geographic information systems (GIS) can help map underserved areas, while health information systems (HIS) track patient access patterns and outcomes [46, 47]. Evidence-based decision-making relies on these data points to guide resource allocation, target interventions to high-need populations, and tailor programs to local contexts [48]. Furthermore, real-time data can be used to detect emerging challenges and adapt strategies dynamically.

7.3 Continuous quality improvement in healthcare access strategies

Healthcare access strategies must be flexible and continuously improved to remain effective.

Continuous quality improvement (CQI) methodologies, such as the Plan-Do-Study-Act (PDSA) cycle, help ensure that healthcare initiatives evolve to meet changing community needs [49]. CQI involves ongoing evaluation of interventions, collecting feedback from stakeholders, and adjusting strategies based on performance metrics and outcome data [50]. This iterative approach fosters innovation in service delivery models, such as telemedicine and mobile clinics, and strengthens the sustainability of healthcare programs. Additionally, engaging frontline healthcare workers and community members in the CQI process helps identify practical solutions to access barriers, ensuring more responsive and locally relevant interventions [51].

8. Conclusion

This chapter provides a robust foundation for understanding the complexities of healthcare access and outlines evidence-based strategies necessary for its improvement. By focusing on policy and regulatory measures, healthcare access can be expanded across diverse populations and settings, addressing the systemic gaps that prevent equitable care.

Improving healthcare infrastructure is key to ensuring more equitable access, particularly in underserved areas where facilities and resources are often lacking. Building healthcare capacity, along with the introduction of telemedicine, mobile clinics, and outreach programs, brings essential services closer to the people who need them most.

Financial strategies, such as subsidies, sliding fee scales, and the reduction of out-of-pocket expenses, are crucial in breaking down the economic barriers that often prevent individuals from seeking care. These measures help ensure that healthcare is affordable and accessible for all, regardless of socioeconomic status.

Workforce development and distribution strategies, including training, task-shifting, and incentivizing healthcare professionals to serve in rural and underserved areas, are essential in addressing healthcare shortages. By enhancing the skills and distribution of healthcare workers, these strategies ensure that quality care reaches marginalized populations.

Community engagement and advocacy further support the goal of improved healthcare access by involving local populations in decision-making and empowering them to advocate for their healthcare rights.

Grassroots movements and initiatives create a more inclusive healthcare system that responds to the specific needs of diverse communities.

Finally, continuous monitoring and evaluation are vital for refining healthcare access strategies. By measuring the impact of interventions and using data to guide improvement efforts, healthcare systems can make informed adjustments that lead to lasting improvements in access for all populations.

Acknowledgements

The present book chapter was not funded institutionally or by anyone else.

Conflict of interest

The authors declare no competing interests.

Acronyms and abbreviations

ACA	affordable care act
LMICs	low- and middle-income countries

NGOs	non-governmental organizations
OOP	out-of-pocket
CHWs	community health workers
M&E	monitoring and evaluation
RE-AIM model	reach, effectiveness, adoption, implementation, and maintenance
GIS	geographic information systems
HIS	health information systems
CQI	continuous quality improvement
PDSA	plan-do-study-act

Author details

Feyissa Regassa Senbato[1*], Deneke Wolde[2], Kasu T. Bifa[3] and Tesfaye G. Bikila[1]

1 Addis Ababa University College of Health Science Tikur Anbessa Specialized Hospital Addis Ababa, Ethiopia

2 Department of Medical Laboratory Science, College of Medicine and Health Sciences, Wachemo University, Hossana, Ethiopia

3 Ministry of Health Addis Ababa, Ethiopia

*Address all correspondence to: feyissa.regassa@aau.edu.et

References

[1] WHO. WHO Global Strategy on Health, Environment and Climate Change the Transformation Needed to Improve Lives and Well Being Sustainably through Healthy Environments. Switzerland: World Health Organization; 2020

[2] Gurewich D, Garg A, Kressin NR. Addressing social determinants of health within healthcare delivery systems: A framework to ground and inform health outcomes. Journal of General Internal Medicine. 2020;**35**:1571-1575. DOI: 10.1007/s11606-020-05720-6

[3] Shrank WH, Deparle NA, Gottlieb S, Jain SH, Orszag P, Powers BW, et al. Health costs and financing: Challenges and strategies for a new administration. Health Affairs. 2021;**40**:235-242. DOI: 10.1377/hlthaff.2020.01560

[4] Vart P. Understanding the social determinants of health. The Lancet. 2022;**399**:1467. DOI: 10.1016/S0140-6736(21)02660-X

[5] Honein MA, Christie A, Rose DA, Brooks JT, Meaney-Delman D, Cohn A, et al. Summary of guidance for public health strategies to address high levels of community transmission of SARS-CoV-2 and related deaths. In: Morbidity and Mortality Weekly Report. United States; 2020

[6] Evans MV, Andréambeloson T, Randriamihaja M, Ihantamalala F, Cordier L, Cowley G, et al. Geographic barriers to care persist at the community healthcare level: Evidence from rural Madagascar. PLOS Global Public Health. 2022;**2**:9-11. DOI: 10.1371/journal.pgph.0001028

[7] Al Shamsi H, Almutairi AG, Al Mashrafi S, Al KT. Implications of language barriers for healthcare: A systematic review. Oman Medical Journal. 2020;**35**:1-7. DOI: 10.5001/OMJ.2020.40

[8] Oleribe OO, Momoh J, Uzochukwu BSC, Mbofana F, Adebiyi A, Barbera T, et al. Identifying key challenges facing healthcare systems in Africa and potential solutions. International Journal of General Medicine. 2019;**12**:395-403. DOI: 10.2147/IJGM.S223882

[9] Jia L, Yuan B, Huang F, Lu Y, Garner P, Meng Q. Strategies for expanding health insurance coverage in vulnerable populations. Cochrane Database of Systematic Reviews. 2014;**2014**:395-403. DOI: 10.1002/14651858.CD008194.pub3

[10] Semprini J, Lyu W, Shane DM, Wehby GL. The effects of ACA medicaid expansions on health after 5 years. Medical Care Research and Review. 2022;**79**:28-35. DOI: 10.1177/1077558720972592

[11] Barker AR, Li L. The cumulative impact of health insurance on health status. Health Services Research (United States). 2020;**55**:815-822. DOI: 10.1111/1475-6773.13325

[12] Linda Luxon. Infrastructure—The Key to Healthcare Improvement. 2015

[13] Vincent RS. The high cost of prescription drugs: Causes and solutions. Blood Cancer Journal. 2020;**10**:815-822. DOI: 10.1038/s41408-020-0338-x

[14] Claire Borelli M, Bujanda M, Maier K. The affordable care act insurance reforms: Where are we now, and what's next? Clinical

Diabetes. 2016;**34**:58-64. DOI: 10.2337/diaclin.34.1.58

[15] Field MJ, Lohr KN, Yordy KD. Assessing Health Care Reform. United States: National Academy Press; 1993

[16] Edgman-Levitan S, Schoenbaum SC. Patient-centered care: Achieving higher quality by designing care through the patient's eyes. Israel Journal Health Policy Research. 2021;**10**:54. DOI: 10.1186/s13584-021-00459-9

[17] Gizaw Z, Astale T, Kassie GM. What improves access to primary healthcare services in rural communities? A systematic review. BMC Primary Care (Ethiopia). 2022;**23**:2-5. DOI: 10.1186/s12875-022-01919-0

[18] WHO. Who Guidance for Climate-Resilient and Environmentally Sustainable Health Care Facilities. 2020

[19] Haleem A, Javaid M, Singh RP, Suman R. Telemedicine for healthcare: Capabilities, features, barriers, and applications. Sensors International. 2021;**2**:27. DOI: 10.1016/j.sintl.2021.100117

[20] Hollander JE, Carr BG. Virtually perfect? Telemedicine for Covid-19. New England Journal of Medicine. 2020;**382**:1679-1681. DOI: 10.1056/nejmp2003539

[21] Singh S, Baig F, Singh S. Mobile health clinics as a healthcare delivery model to address community disparities. Kansas Journal of Medicine (United States). 2022;**15**:259-261. DOI: 10.17161/kjm.vol15.16543

[22] WHO. Community-Based Health Care, Including Outreach and Campaigns, in the Context of the COVID-19 Pandemic Interim Guidance. 2020

[23] Idriss-Wheeler D, Ormel I, Assefa M, Rab F, Angelakis C, Yaya S, et al. Engaging community health workers (CHWs) in Africa: Lessons from the Canadian red cross supported programs. PLOS Global Public Health. 2024;**4**:63-69. DOI: 10.1371/journal.pgph.0002799

[24] Dawkins B, Renwick C, Ensor T, Shinkins B, Jayne D, Meads D. What factors affect patients' ability to access healthcare? An overview of systematic reviews. Tropical Medicine and International Health. 2021;**26**:1177-1188. DOI: 10.1111/tmi.13651

[25] Bou-Karroum L, Iaia DG, El-Jardali F, Abou Samra C, Salameh S, Sleem Z, et al. Financing for equity for women's, children's and adolescents' health in low- and middle-income countries: A scoping review. PLOS Global Public Health. 2024;**4**:e0003573. DOI: 10.1371/journal.pgph.0003573

[26] Asante A, Price J, Hayen A, Jan S, Wiseman V. Equity in health care financing in low-and middle-income countries: A systematic review of evidence from studies using benefit and financing incidence analyses. PLoS One (Ghana). 2016;**11**:15-18. DOI: 10.1371/journal.pone.0152866

[27] Rochelle E. Dahmen. Sliding Fee Scale Discount Guide for Critical Access Hospitals and Rural Health Clinics. 2022

[28] Sturmberg JP, Bircher J. Better and fulfilling healthcare at lower costs: The need to manage health systems as complex adaptive systems. F1000Res. 2019;**8**:8-9. DOI: 10.12688/F1000RESEARCH.19414.1

[29] Jalali FS, Bikineh P, Delavari S. Strategies for reducing out of pocket payments in the health system: A scoping review. Cost Effectiveness and

Resource Allocation. 2021;**19**:235-242. DOI: 10.1186/s12962-021-00301-8

[30] Russell D, Mathew S, Fitts M, Liddle Z, Murakami-Gold L, Campbell N, et al. Interventions for health workforce retention in rural and remote areas: A systematic review. Human Resources for Health (Australia). 2021;**19**:8-9. DOI: 10.1186/s12960-021-00643-7

[31] Strasser R, Neusy AJ. De l'importance du contexte: La formation de professionnels de la santé dans et pour les zones rurales et isolées. Bulletin of the World Health Organization. 2010;**88**:777-782. DOI: 10.2471/BLT.09.072462

[32] WHO. WHO Guideline on Health Policy and System Support to Optimize Community Health Worker Programmes. 2018

[33] Ahmed S, Chase LE, Wagnild J, Akhter N, Sturridge S, Clarke A, et al. Community health workers and health equity in low- and middle-income countries: Systematic review and recommendations for policy and practice. International Journal for Equity in Health. 2022;**21**:777-782. DOI: 10.1186/s12939-021-01615-y

[34] Bärnighausen T, Bloom DE. Financial incentives for return of service in underserved areas: A systematic review. BMC Health Services Research. 2009;**9**:57-60. DOI: 10.1186/1472-6963-9-86

[35] Dolea C, Stormont L, Braichet JM. Evaluated strategies to increase attraction and retention of health workers in remote and rural areas. Bulletin of the World Health Organization. 2010;**88**:379-385. DOI: 10.2471/BLT.09.070607

[36] Rifkin SB. Examining the links between community participation and health outcomes: A review of the literature. Health Policy and Planning. 2014;**29**:ii98-i106. DOI: 10.1093/heapol/czu076

[37] Morales-Garzón S, Parker LA, Hernández-Aguado I, González-Moro Tolosana M, Pastor-Valero M, Chilet-Rosell E. Addressing health disparities through community participation: A scoping review of co-creation in public health. Healthcare (Switzerland). 2023;**11**:379-385. DOI: 10.3390/healthcare11071034

[38] Draper AK, Rifkin SB. Community Participation in Health Systems Development. Achieving Person-Centred Health Systems: Evidence, Strategies and Challenges. United States: Cambridge University Press; 2020. pp. 115-143. DOI: 10.1017/9781108855464.008

[39] Haldane V, Chuah FLH, Srivastava A, Singh SR, Koh GCH, Seng CK, et al. Community participation in health services development, implementation, and evaluation: A systematic review of empowerment, health, community, and process outcomes. PLoS One. (Singapore). 2019;**14**:16. DOI: 10.1371/journal.pone.0216112

[40] Myers CR. Promoting population health: Nurse advocacy, policy making, and use of media. Nursing Clinics of North America. 2020;**55**:11-20. DOI: 10.1016/j.cnur.2019.11.001

[41] World Health Organization (WHO). Framework on Integrated, People-Centred Health Services Report by the Secretariat. Switzerland; 2016

[42] Friedman LS, SB. Models of population health: Their value for US public health practice, policy, and research. American Journal of Public Health (United States). 2003;**93**:366-369. DOI: 10.2105/ajph.93.3.366

[43] Bhutta ZA, Lassi ZS, Pariyo G, Huicho L. Global Evidence of Community Health Workers Global Experience of Community Health Workers for Delivery of Health Related Millennium Development Goals: A Systematic Review, Country Case Studies, and Recommendations for Integration into National Health Systems. Switzerland: World Health Organization (WHO); 2013

[44] Finley EP, Moore G, Yuan S, Glasgow RE. Use of the Reach, Effectiveness, Adoption, Implementation, and Maintenance (RE-AIM) Framework to Guide Iterative Adaptations: Applications, Lessons Learned, and Future Directions. United States; 2022

[45] Clarke GM, Conti S, Wolters AT, Steventon A. Evaluating the impact of healthcare interventions using routine data. The BMJ. 2019;**365**:117-118. DOI: 10.1136/bmj.l2239

[46] Nykiforuk CIJ, Flaman LM. Geographic information systems (GIS) for health promotion and public health: A review. Health Promotion Practice. 2011;**12**:63-73. DOI: 10.1177/1524839909334624

[47] Fletcher-Lartey SM, Caprarelli G. Application of GIS technology in public health: Successes and challenges. Parasitology. 2016;**143**:401-415. DOI: 10.1017/S0031182015001869

[48] Shafaghat T, Bastani P, Nasab MHI, Bahrami MA, Montazer MRA, Zarchi MKR, et al. A framework of evidence-based decision-making in health system management: A best-fit framework synthesis. Archives of Public Health. 2022;**80**:63-73. DOI: 10.1186/s13690-022-00843-0

[49] Hill JE, Stephani AM, Sapple P, Clegg AJ. The effectiveness of continuous quality improvement for developing professional practice and improving health care outcomes: A systematic review. Implementation Science. 2020;**15**:401-415. DOI: 10.1186/s13012-020-0975-2

[50] Endalamaw A, Khatri RB, Mengistu TS, Erku D, Wolka E, Zewdie A, et al. A scoping review of continuous quality improvement in healthcare system: Conceptualization, models and tools, barriers and facilitators, and impact. BMC Health Services Research. 2024;**24**:5-6. DOI: 10.1186/s12913-024-10828-0

[51] Needleman J, Pearson ML, Upenieks VV, Yee T, Wolstein J, Parkerton M. Engaging frontline staff in performance improvement: The American Organization of Nurse Executives implementation of transforming care at the bedside collaborative. Joint Commission Journal on Quality and Patient Safety. 2016;**42**:61-69. DOI: 10.1016/s1553-7250(16)42007-6

Chapter 2

Perspective Chapter: An Exploration of Provider Access, Cost and Quality Impacting the Total Cost of Healthcare for Employers in the United States

Ronald J. Ozminkowski, Wendy M. Smith, Weiyee Lee, Phil Salinger, Pedro Jofre Lora, Brandon Young and Sandip Gupta

Abstract

Many factors can positively or negatively influence access to healthcare, depending on whether or how they are managed. Our new Health Equity and Affordability Tool (HEAT) leverages 59 machine learning models to show employers and other health insurance carriers how access problems relate to individuals' healthcare affordability and whether they reside in areas with shortages of primary care and mental health providers. HEAT also shows how access relates to local healthcare provider costs and quality of care. The insights provided then illustrate how access to less costly and higher quality care can be enhanced. For this chapter, HEAT was used to illustrate the above for an employer client and how that client's characteristics compared to other clients in the same industry. Results showed that 23% of the client's insured members spend more than 10% of their income in healthcare. Also, two-thirds of insured employees live in areas with high shortages of mental health providers. Affordability varied significantly by gender, and quality of care differed greatly across the region. Remedies to these problems might include steerage to lower cost providers, offering virtual care in areas of shortage, and providing self-service tools to find lower cost and higher quality providers.

Keywords: access, equity, quality of care, cost of care, healthcare affordability, insurance, chronic condition prevalence, healthcare utilization, health plan features, out-of-pocket costs, work time loss, healthcare claims

1. Introduction

Many macroeconomic factors such as anti-competitive market practices, healthcare price inflation, and provider shortages are creating challenges for employers related to healthcare costs, affordability and equity. For example, by 2028 Aon analyses of Bureau of Labor Statistics [1] data project that 41% of employer spending on "total rewards" (e.g., wages, benefits, bonuses, stock, etc.) will come from their contributions to employee benefits. They also project that the increases in the healthcare costs employers pay will be more than twice what they pay for retirement or paid leave benefits, and more than three times the increases in wages they expect to pay. Healthcare cost increases by 2028 also are expected to be about four times as high as the 9% level of general inflation measured in early 2024.

Ever increasing healthcare costs also pose problems for individual consumers. According to the Commonwealth Fund Survey of Health Insurance [2], 68% of people with incomes less than twice the federal poverty level were unable to pay $1000 for an unexpected medical bill in 2022, as were 69% of Black survey respondents and 63% of Hispanic respondents. About 42% of white respondents were unable to pay $1000 for an unexpected medical bill as well. These individuals are assumed to be "functionally underinsured."

Also, according to the Kaiser Family Foundation [3], 59% of women have difficulty affording their bills each month, compared to 39% of men, but men were more likely to delay care or to seek care with more severe conditions than were women.

Healthcare cost increases influence access to care as well. About 32% of respondents to the 2022 Commonwealth Fund [2] survey reported access problems due to high healthcare costs, as did 61% of the functionally underinsured respondents. Competing pressures coming from increasing food and fuel prices and housing or rent prices may force tradeoffs between healthcare and other basic needs.

It is important to be specific when talking about access to care because it has many dimensions and may mean different things to consumers, providers, policy makers, or payers [4, 5]. The access determinants we focus on in this chapter pertain to healthcare affordability, equity, limited local supplies of primary care and mental health providers, increasing market concentration of providers, and other cost- and quality-related factors that influence the ability to obtain healthcare.

For example, **Table 1** shows results from an analysis of orthopedic surgeons in Dallas, Texas, conducted by Garner Health [6], revealed significant variability in complication rates post-surgery across all major healthcare systems. The study found that within the same healthcare system, some doctors exhibited complication rates more than three times higher than their high-performing peers. Although high-performing doctors are accessible to the majority of patients, the primary challenge lies in identifying these top-performing physicians with the limited resources currently available to consumers. The table below shows a sample of ten of these providers and their widely varying complications rates.

Employers can use several tools to address relationships between access, quality of care, equity, and healthcare costs. According to the 2024 Aon Health Survey [7], about 35% of employers increased efforts to steer insured members to higher-quality and/or more cost-effective hospitals. Over a quarter of surveyed employers provided a self-service cost and quality transparency tool in 2024, and 24% tailored cost-sharing requirements based upon selection of providers and/or particular treatment options. Incentives to improve access for underserved members can be provided within these options and others described below.

For any particular employer, approaches to improve access, equity, quality and reduce costs are likely to vary according to how problematic these factors

Garner's dataset in greater Dallas contains data on:		Complications following joint replacement				
		Doctor	**Hospital(s)**	**Surgeries**	**Complications**	**Complication Rate**
		Dr. F	BSW	388	35	9%
		Dr. D.	**BSW**	**171**	**16**	**9%**
7.1 m	Patients	Dr. D.	Texas Health	321	30	9%
		Dr. S.	BSW	788	73	9%
		Dr. A.	BSW	204	20	10%
51.8 k	Providers	Dr. C.	Methodist	408	114	28%
386.7 m	Claims	Dr. F.	BSW	292	82	28%
		Dr. R.	Texas Health	1428	407	29%
		Dr. E.	Texas Health	1914	547	29%
		Dr. R.	BSW	1963	593	30%
garner™		Dallas Metro Area		35,328	1308	16%

Table 1.
Complications.

are among their insured members. Below we describe how a new Health Equity and Affordability Tool (HEAT) provides estimates of the magnitude of problems related to:

- healthcare affordability,
- social determinants of health (SDOH),
- shortages of primary care and mental health providers,
- increasing market concentration, gender inequities, and
- limited supplies of high-quality/low-cost providers within the insured network.

We focus primarily on access, quality, and cost relationships and illustrate what employers can do to remedy the problems they face.

2. Access, health equity, and affordability tools

2.1 Heat overview

As shown in **Figure 1**, the HEAT is a free analytic solution developed in 2022 and updated recently for 2024. Since its inception until the time of this writing, HEAT has been used 996 times on behalf of 754 Aon clients.

The 2022 version provided employers with insights related to healthcare affordability, SDOH, and access to primary care and mental health providers. Information about hospital market concentration and provider cost and quality were added in

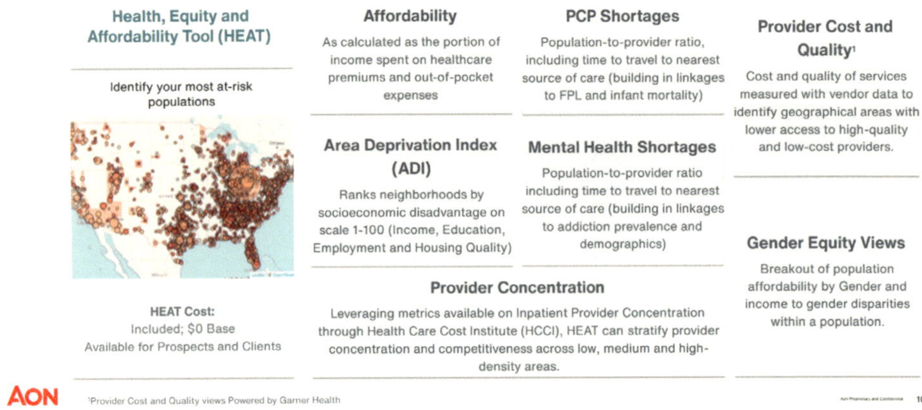

Figure 1.
Understanding health equity and affordability gaps across an insured population.

the 2024 release. HEAT can show how these relate to each other for a client's insured members overall and by gender. HEAT also provides benchmarks about these issues for 12 industry categories[1] based upon information from 517 companies ranging from 62 to 539,902 covered lives.

As noted in Section 3 below, HEAT dashboards show predicted outcomes related to health plan design, chronic condition prevalence, healthcare utilization, behavioral habits, and time lost from work. HEAT shows how these are in turn related to healthcare affordability, SDOH, and the availability, cost, and quality of services from local healthcare providers. These are all components of a well-rounded conceptual model of access to healthcare such as that described in seminal work by Penchansky and Thomas [4].

The outcomes shown in HEAT are provided on separate views for the index categories shown in the boxes of **Figure 1** above. For each of these index categories, HEAT provides views that cover all employees. HEAT also can generate information separately for males and females and for varying levels of family income.

Maps such as the one shown in **Figure 1** are included for each index category in HEAT as well. Hovering over any of the colored circles on these maps will provide information about the number of employees an employer or prospect has in the county of interest where employees live. Color coding for the counties on the maps refer to low, medium, or high average levels of risk for each index category, for employees who live there.

The maps and other visuals shown in HEAT were developed using Shiny by R [8].

For provider cost and quality metrics, the HEAT tool utilizes data provided by Garner Health, a leading healthcare data company that offers both analytical insights and employer solutions. Garner defines quality based on a physician's adherence to the published clinical literature pertinent to their specialty. Practically, this adherence translates to the avoidance of unnecessary procedures, complex imaging, and inappropriate prescriptions.

1 Industry categories include Agriculture, Forestry, and Fishing; Construction; Energy, Utilities, and Mining; Entertainment and Leisure; Finance and Insurance; Healthcare; Manufacturing; Professional Services; Public Sector; Retail and Wholesale Trade; Technology and Communications; and Transportation.

The cost associated with a physician is influenced by their negotiated procedural rates, the frequency of utilizing high-cost service sites, and the affiliated facilities commonly used for major procedures. Garner's rankings reflect the overall cost and quality of providers across different geographic areas, indicating what percentage of the population has access to top-tier providers in their region.

Significant disparities exist between the cost and quality of care patients currently receive and the superior care available from the highest-performing doctors in their vicinity.

Within the HEAT Tool, Garner's data is aggregated at the county level, providing a layered analysis over the locations of a client's insured population.

The HEAT tool itself is not released directly to clients. Aon account executives and consultants provide a visual display of the tool in a video call with the client. After that call, the client receives an Export Report which summarizes results from the HEAT run. Several of the views from the Export Report are shown below.

3. An application

Access barriers are not just mere inconveniences which delay necessary medical care. Whether those barriers are due to the high costs of care or underinsurance which makes it unaffordable, or other issues such as lacking a usual source of care, limited availability or accessibility of care, racism or other discrimination [9], delays can be deadly. For example, Prentice and Pizer [10] found that patients who had to wait longer than 31 days for care at a geriatric outpatient clinic operated by a Veterans Administration medical center in the United States (U.S.) were 21% more likely to die, compared to Veterans who were able to receive care faster.

Moreover, greater access to care does not always mean having access to higher-quality providers. Asch, et al. [11] showed that just under 55% of adults in the 12 communities they studied did not receive all the care recommended for their problems. Percentages varied slightly yet significantly by race and income, though all percentages were below 60%. In addition, poor access due to lower affordability is associated with increases in hospitalization [3]. Also, poor access due to living in an underserved community has been associated with higher rates of diabetes and cardiovascular disease, as well as earlier death [12].

HEAT has been designed to show relationships between affordability, living in underserved areas due to socioeconomic or health care supply limitations, chronic condition prevalence, health plan design features, behavioral habits and risks, and time lost from work. The following excerpts from a HEAT Export Report illustrate these relationships.

Figure 2 shows a HEAT output for several companies working in the Agriculture, Forestry, and Fishing Industry. As shown in the bar chart there, about 47% of employees had medium levels of affordability, meaning they spent between 5% and 10% of their family incomes on healthcare. About 30% had high affordability, meaning they spent less than 5% of their incomes on healthcare, and just over 23% had low affordability, spending more than 10% of their incomes on healthcare. Employers in this industry (or elsewhere) might wish to consider plan design, subsidies, referrals to lower-cost providers, or other remedies to reduce affordability problems.

The text comment above the bar chart on **Figure 2** also shows how one simulated company in the Agriculture, Forestry, and Fishing industry compared to all

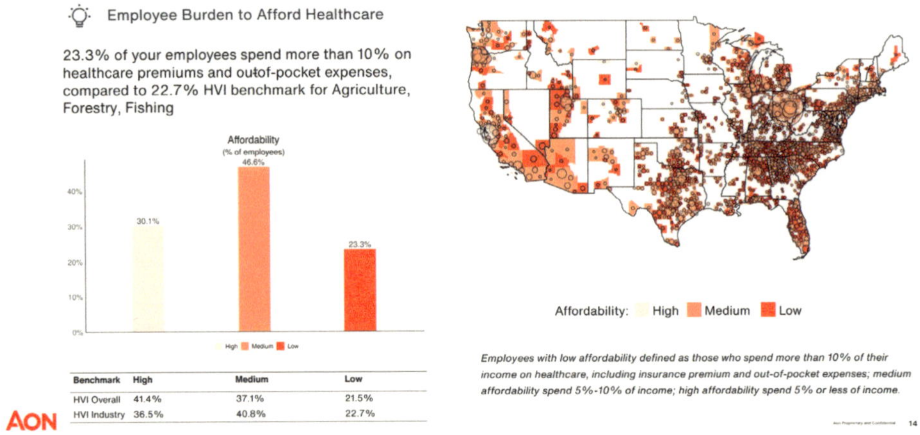

Figure 2.
Affordability.

companies in the HEAT data set and in that industry. Differences in affordability are not stark in this case, but since all companies had nearly 22% in the low affordability group, leaders may still be advised to consider affordability remedies.

Finally, the map on the right in the figure shows the distribution of people in the affordability groups in locations where these companies have employees.

Next, **Figure 3** shows how affordability varies by income and gender for the same company and industry group. Differences between males and females may be affected by the Gender Inequity factors listed on the right side of the figure. Strategies to reduce gender differences might include greater equity regarding maternal and paternal leave benefits, better fertility of adoption benefits for each gender, strengthening benefits to address same-sex-partner- or gender-transition- health coverage, and better access for treating mental health problems that tend to affect genders differently.

Moving on, **Figure 4** shows differences in problems related to SDOH, as measured by the Area Deprivation Index (ADI), which measures barriers to healthcare associated with the neighborhoods where people live[2]. This view was again created for one client in the Agriculture, Forestry, and Fishing industry, but similar views can be shown for other industries or for other individual companies. For this industry and client, substantially fewer of the insureds fell into the Low ADI group, and many more fell into the High ADI group, compared to companies in all industries (see the comment at the top of the bar chart and the table at bottom it in the **Figure 4**). The map at the right in the figure shows how ADI average scores vary by county across the country for that industry group.

[2] The Area Deprivation Index was created originally by the federal Health Resources and Services Administration and then moved to the University of Wisconsin's Neighborhood Atlas website [13] where data from 2015–2022 are available. ADI values range from 0 to 100, with higher scores indicating greater problems related to social determinants of health. For our analyses, living in an area where the ADI value was less than or equal to 33 indicated living in a low-risk ADI area, representing few barriers related to social determinants of health. ADI scores ranging from 33-66 indicated living in a medium-risk ADI area, where those barriers were somewhat greater. ADI scores above 66 indicated living in a high-risk ADI area, where barriers related to social determinants of health were the greatest.

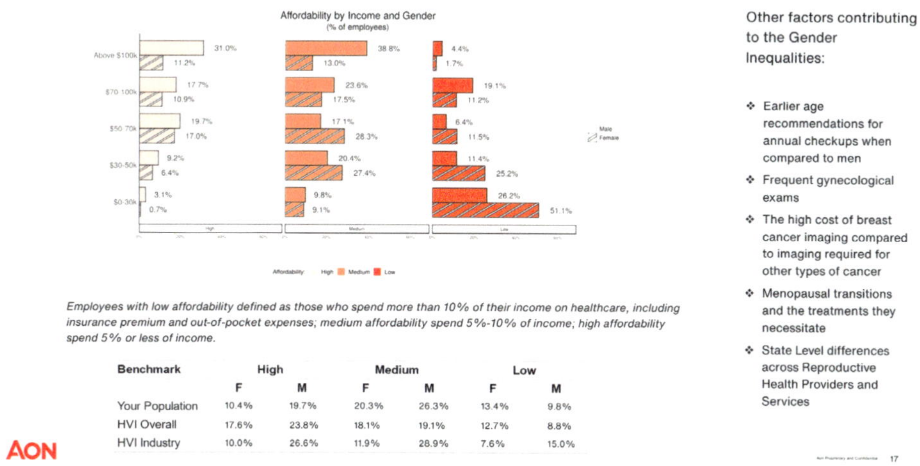

Figure 3.
Health affordability by income and gender.

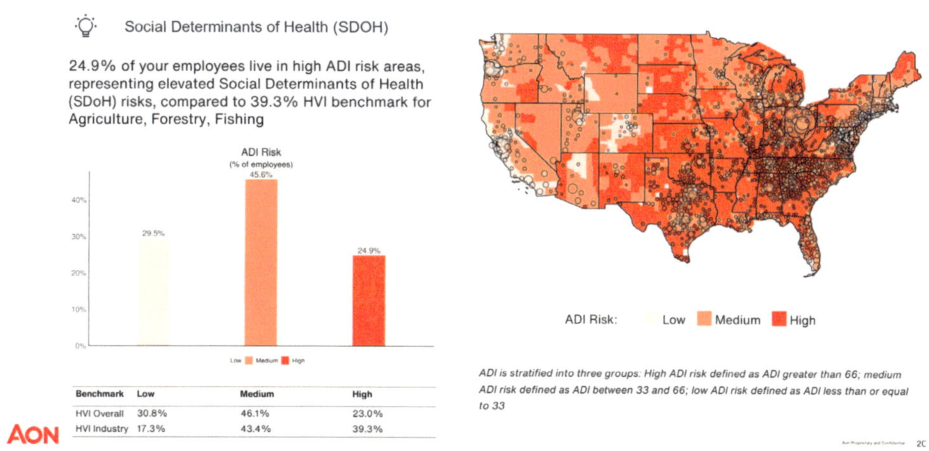

Figure 4.
Area deprivation index (ADI) and SDOH differences.

The ADI score ranges shown in **Figure 4** range from 0 to 100, with higher scores illustrating greater problems receiving health care. These can be due to geographic access problems, transportation barriers, poor education, limited supplies of medical specialists, or other factors.

Remedies for ADI-related problems might include offering wellbeing programs as an employee benefit, for free or at low cost. Other potential remedies include providing telehealth or travel benefits so workers and family members can gain access to lower-cost or higher-quality providers, and offering enhanced care management programs that link individuals to many different types of social agencies which can address problems that also have implications related to poor health. Ozminkowski and

Metcalfe [14] provide information on how employers can work with many partners to enhance management of medical, social, judicial, and other problems.

Next, many employees live in areas where there are shortages of primary care or mental health providers. HEAT output for the Agriculture, Forestry, and Fishing industry show that about 34% of employees live in areas of high primary care physician shortages, while almost two-thirds (65.7%) live in areas with high shortages of mental health providers. Potential remedies for these problems include virtual primary care or urgent care offered by external partners. State or federal subsidies should also be considered, as these are widespread national problems in the U.S.

Also, empirical evidence shows that about 75% of the inpatient hospital markets in the U.S. are highly concentrated or may become so, meaning that hospitals tend to be owned by only one or a small number of health systems [15]. Highly concentrated markets can lead to access problems when older, less profitable facilities are closed by new owners as the market consolidates. Research also suggests that consolidation often leads to higher prices for care, causing access problems that exacerbate affordability issues [12].

HEAT results for the client company and the Agriculture, Forestry, and Fishing Industry contrast with the 75% figure mentioned above, however. **Figure 5** shows that only about 22% of the insureds in that industry who work for Aon clients live in highly consolidated areas. About 40% of the insureds from the client company live in highly consolidated areas. For some of these people, higher prices due to consolidated market power might pose access problems related to lower affordability.

Some potential remedies that might help people who live in more highly consolidated areas were mentioned by respondents to the 2024 Aon Employer Health Survey [6]. These include providing a self-service cost and quality transparency tool, which was cited by 52% of respondents, either as part of their 2024 plan, or as something they are interested in adding. Similar, working with external navigation partners to guide people to lower-cost and/or better providers was cited by 49% of respondents. Narrowing health insurance network choices to focus more on lower-cost or higher-quality providers was either being used or planned by 38% of respondents, but the

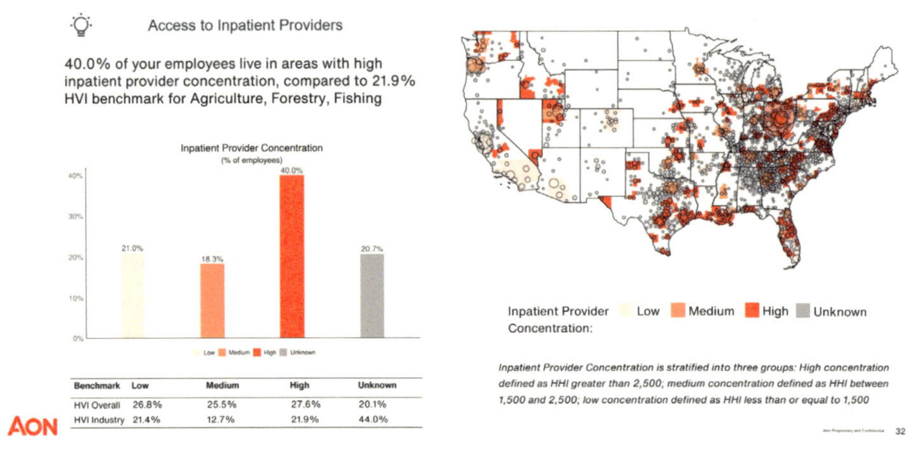

Figure 5.
Inpatient provider concentration.

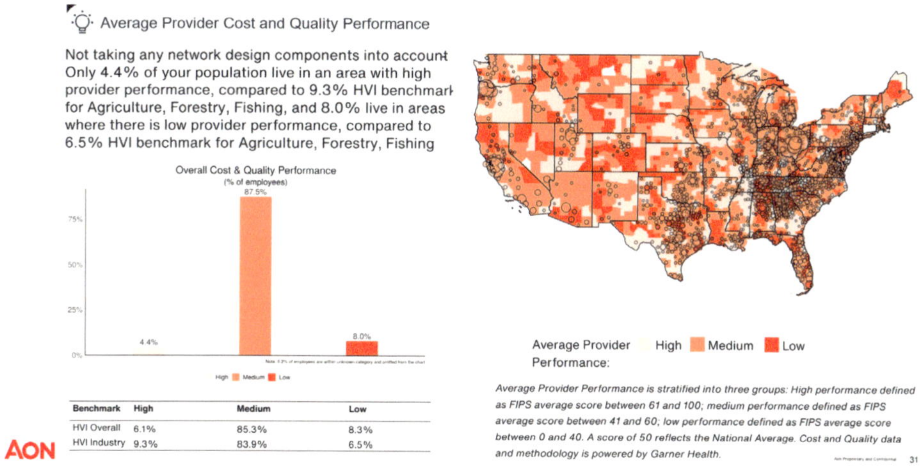

Benchmark	High	Medium	Low
HVI Overall	6.1%	85.3%	8.3%
HVI Industry	9.3%	83.9%	6.5%

Figure 6.
Provider cost and quality.

impact of this policy should be evaluated to learn whether it poses other access-related problems.

The story of healthcare provider cost and quality is a little different. **Figure 6** summarizes provider cost and quality metrics for the client company, the Agriculture, Forestry, and Fishing industry, and for all clients in the HEAT data base. As with the ADI analysis mentioned earlier, cost and quality scores range from 0 to 100. These were calculated by Garner Health after reviewing patterns of care inferred from reviews of over 500 quality criteria applied to over 60 billion health insurance claims.

Two interesting issues were observed about cost and quality when this analysis was conducted:

- First, the pattern shown by the bar chart in **Figure 6** for the Agriculture, Forestry, and Fishing industry was very similar to results calculated separately for each of the other 11 industries.

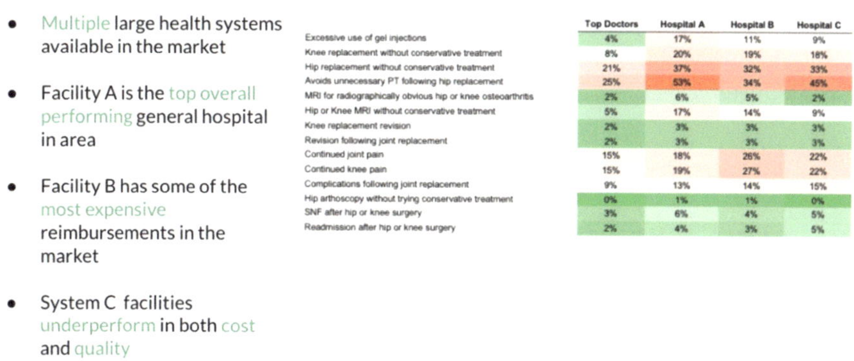
Multiple large health systems available in the market
Facility A is the top overall performing general hospital in area
Facility B has some of the most expensive reimbursements in the market
System C facilities underperform in both cost and quality

	Top Doctors	Hospital A	Hospital B	Hospital C
Excessive use of gel injections	4%	17%	11%	9%
Knee replacement without conservative treatment	8%	20%	19%	18%
Hip replacement without conservative treatment	21%	37%	32%	33%
Avoids unnecessary PT following hip replacement	25%	53%	34%	45%
MRI for radiographically obvious hip or knee osteoarthritis	2%	6%	5%	2%
Hip or Knee MRI without conservative treatment	5%	17%	14%	9%
Knee replacement revision	2%	3%	3%	3%
Revision following joint replacement	2%	3%	3%	3%
Continued joint pain	15%	18%	26%	22%
Continued knee pain	15%	19%	27%	22%
Complications following joint replacement	9%	13%	14%	15%
Hip arthoscopy without trying conservative treatment	0%	1%	1%	0%
SNF after hip or knee surgery	3%	6%	4%	5%
Readmission after hip or knee surgery	2%	4%	3%	5%

Figure 7.
A closer look at hospital systems in your market.

- Second, relatively few people live in areas where the overall average cost and quality performance was either low or high, while over 80% live in areas of medium performance.

Specific to provider cost and quality, there are additional deliverables produced by Garner to supplement the readily available county-level data that is showcased in HEAT.

As noted in **Figure 7**, Garner produces market-specific views that help showcase facility performance in any given geographic area, emphasizing top-performing facilities and the components of cost and quality that drive and support those scores.

Zooming in one level farther, Garner can also produce reports that identify top-performing individual physicians within those hospital systems based on cost and quality performance.

4. What happens next?

Employers will be more educated on access, affordability, and provider costs and quality as data sources are layered such that a visualization tells the story. By combining layering the data from Aon's HEAT tool with 60 million patient lines measured by Garner Health analytics, Employers can make sense of the data visualization outputs focused on the Affordability Index, SDOH, Provider Concentrations, and metrics that score Provider Quality. This is powerful and empowering information that allow for better carrier network choice, alignment for additional services where there are access and affordability issues. Layering these data sources is critical to understanding the magnitude of issues their employees must overcome.

A robust framework must also facilitate actionable opportunities that enhance outcomes over time. Aon and Garner collaborate with their mutual clients under a comprehensive "Discover, Advise, Solution" framework.

Figure 8 shows that insights generated from the HEAT tool enable employers to identify at-risk populations across various categories. Garner's reporting refines these insights, pinpointing specific specialties and markets while highlighting potential provider cost and quality disparities. Upon discovering these insights, Aon and Garner partner to offer consulting on actionable opportunities. They thoroughly understand the current state of medical costs and quality, advising employers on tailored solutions.

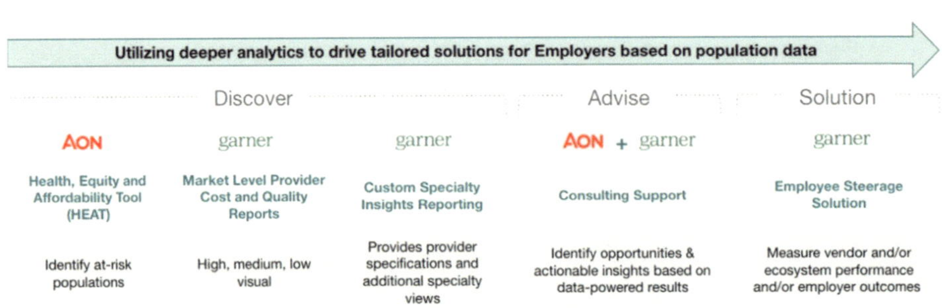

Figure 8.
Using HEAT with additional analytics of population data to address care access, quality, and cost challenges.

There are numerous methods to address challenges related to provider access, cost, and quality. Some approaches focus on physically facilitating member access to physicians. Solutions may include funding ride-sharing services to transport members to qualified physicians, establishing employer-funded clinics in areas with limited access, or creating temporary mobile care sites.

Another set of approaches concentrates on specific specialties, such as mental health, primary care, or women's health, aiming to remove obstacles to generalist care and improve overall access. Additionally, certain solutions utilize overall plan design and transparency tools to help members locate and utilize superior physicians. The optimal solution depends on the nature of the risk, available resources, and the employer's operational capacity.

In particular, the third category of plan design and benefit changes can be implemented using various incentives. A stringent example might involve narrowing the network to include only high-quality providers. Although this could strongly incentivize the use of top facilities, it may present logistical complexities and potentially provoke negative employee reactions.

Employers evaluating solutions should consider:

- Whether the solution requires a significant plan change, such as a shift to a third-party administrator, or can be implemented within the existing network.

- If any plan design changes restrict provider access.

- The impact of the intervention on member satisfaction and continued engagement with the solution.

Garner offers an incentive account providing members with first-dollar reimbursements, contingent on utilizing top providers with favorable cost and quality metrics. This is complemented by digital tools to help members identify affordable options nearby, fostering significant impact.

Regardless of whether an employer adopts the Garner solution, the data derived from HEAT and Garner's market reporting can inform and guide actionable plans. Post-implementation, employers must monitor the strategy's effectiveness, assessing outcomes both at micro and macro levels.

For its clients, Garner tracks the results of interventions, monitoring realized improvements in cost, quality, and satisfaction.

Table 2 illustrates how these results manifest in individual member experiences. Members achieve savings both transactionally and by avoiding unnecessary costs from providers not adhering to standard clinical guidelines. Non-adherence incurs real costs through complications, low-value facility affiliations, and inappropriate care. These individual interactions, across various specialties, cumulatively drive savings for both plans and patients.

Table 3 presents the results from a mutual client of Aon and Garner over the first half of 2024. Consistent tracking and sharing of these results are crucial for employers to continue investing in interventions that enhance access and cost outcomes for their most underserved employees.

Programs like Garner, when combined with accurate insights, can address significant barriers to care for members. Identifying higher quality providers with lower total costs improves overall affordability. Providing digital tools to search for these

On Apr 29, 2024, Dr. Schumann performed a Cataract Removal on your Team Member		
Cost of Cataract Removal	Dr. Schumann	Non-top providers
Physician cost	$679	$742
Facility cost	$1494	$4221
Ancillary cost	$543	$714
Episode impact	—	*$2961*
Appropriateness & Outcomes		
Inappropriate use of cataract removal	22.7%	32.6%
Episode impact	—	*$599*
Complications following cataract surgery	15.8%	25.9%
Episode impact	—	*$203*
Total Savings	**$4180**	

Table 2.
Your team member received high quality care from Dr. Schumann at a lower cost compared to non-top providers.

Specialties	Relationships created	Savings per relationship	Total savings
OBGYN	65	$3130	$203,450
Orthopedics	47	$4270	$200,690
Oncology	22	$9062	$199,364
Primary Care	324	$473	$153,252
Pediatric Internal Medicine	70	$1846	$129,203
General Surgery	15	$8564	$128,460
Cardiology	33	$2797	$92,301
Ophthalmology	23	$2908	$66,884
Gastroenterology	23	$2553	$58,719
Neurology	22	$957	$21,054
General Med Pediatrics	48	$432	$20,736
ENT	12	$1558	$18,696
Other	235	$333	$78,307
Total	**939**	—	**$1,371,116**

Note: The relationships created during the current plan year (January 2024–June 2024): Savings Per Relationship is projected savings derived from research based on the large claims data, comparing costs associated with Tier 1 providers versus average providers.

Table 3.
As a result, aggregating all the individual episodes gives us a sense of the savings impact YTD.

providers enhances accessibility. Higher quality providers generate better health outcomes, including reduced complications.

An incentive account offering first-dollar coverage for using superior doctors significantly lowers members' out-of-pocket expenses, often eliminating the need to pay any deductible.

In addition to reports demonstrating potential cost and quality savings, Garner provides data on realized improvements based on actual claim experience.

5. Conclusions

Employers who have employees scattered across the U.S. and globally have very little insight into the access, affordability, and SDOH they experience. While transparency is improving, there is also no visualization of provider costs and quality unless the employer has access to data sets and tools that pronounce the problem. Solutions such as the HEAT tool and Garner Health are important as employers make their carrier network selections, as they look at point solutions, as they pinpoint real problem areas. Seek out data and challenge your consultants and carriers to provide this important intel.

Conflict of interest

Dr. Ozminkowski and Ms. Lee are employed by Aon plc. Dr. Smith was employed by Aon when HEAT was developed. Mr. Salinger, Mr. Jofre Lora, Mr. Young, and Mr. Gupta are employed by Garner Health, which developed the provider cost and quality metrics used by HEAT. Aon plc and Garner Health are partners in efforts to show HEAT to clients and prospects. This may or may not lead to client-funded work in the future.

The opinions expressed in this chapter are the authors' and may not represent the opinions of Aon plc or Garner Health.

A.Appendix: Data sources, methodological approach, and empirical models and variables for HEATThis appendix describes the data sources and empirical models used to create the HEAT views. It also provides rules about how to assign low-, medium-, or high-risk values to healthcare affordability, challenges related to SDOH, living in areas where there are shortages of primary care or mental health providers, living in areas where inpatient providers are highly concentrated, and measures of provider cost and quality.

Appendix 1. Data sources

Several data sources were used to create HEAT. First, many of the relationships described in HEAT are based on 59 data science models of chronic condition prevalence, health care utilization, and unit costs for healthcare services incurred by over 1.29 million insured individuals throughout the 50 states. Demographic, location, and health-related data for these models came from insurance membership and claims files and pharmaceutical claims files, reflecting the health insurance coverage offered by Aon clients in 2018.

Second, data from the U.S. Health Resources and Services Administration [16] allowed us to determine whether people lived in areas where there were shortages of primary care or mental health providers, which may create access problems.

Third, data obtained from the Neighborhood Atlas [17] maintained by the University of Wisconsin allowed us to determine whether people lived in areas where challenges related to SDOH were great or less problematic.

Fourth, data from the Behavioral Risk Factor Surveillance System [18] surveys for 2016–2020 were used to estimate whether people had problems related to tobacco use, obesity, other nutritional problems, or alcohol use problems.

Finally, demographic and other data were provided by employers or prospects who requested that HEAT be used to create information describing their employees. We refer to data from employers or prospects as census data. These data include employee level measures of age, gender, zip code, salary, bonus payments, insurance coverage type (i.e., employee-only, employee and spouse, family), health plan type (e.g., point of service, preferred provider organization, health maintenance organization, etc.), individual and family coinsurance and deductible requirements, and annual out-of-pocket dollar maximums.

When some employers preferred not to provide salary information, salaries and then family income estimates were imputed based upon other information provided in the census data, along with data science models designed to estimate income that were based on year-2017 Current Population Survey data from the U.S. Bureau of Labor Statistics [13].

Additional information about data file content can be found in Sections 6.3 and 6.4 below.

Appendix 2. Modeling strategy

The underlying strategy for creating the 59 data science models was to generate predictive models of condition prevalence, healthcare utilization, and unit costs, based upon demographic and other information available in the membership and claims files that also could be collected separately from other employer clients or potential clients (i.e., prospects) whose data were not included in the 1.29-million-member sample. Then demographic and other information obtained from these other clients or prospects could be fed into the predictive models created from the analytic files, to generate predictions of prevalence, utilization, and cost that are pertinent to these new clients or prospects.

Appendix 3. Modeling approaches

Modeling with the 1.29-million-member sample data was completed with Python software in a Databricks SDK environment [19].

Our modeling was conducted as follows:

- Logistic regression models were estimated with a backwards selection procedure, to predict the occurrence or not of each of twenty-three[3] chronic conditions, based

[3] The 23 chronic conditions were coded using Clinical Classification Software (CCS) developed by the federal Agency for Healthcare Research and Quality. CCS categories included alcohol use disorders, asthma or chronic obstructive pulmonary disease, high blood pressure, cancers, cardiovascular disorders, diverticulitis, diabetes mellitus, endocrine disorders, esophageal disorders, blood disorders, human immunodeficiency virus, hypothyroid disorder, inflammatory bowel disease, other immune disorders, metabolic disorders, migraine, multiple sclerosis, musculoskeletal disorders (e.g., disk, joint, and arthritis disorders), pregnancy, renal disorders, substance use disorders other than alcohol, and behavioral health disorders (e.g., anxiety, depression, and other mood disorders).

on age, age squared, gender, the ADI of the zip code where each person lived, and interactions between age and ADI, age and gender, and gender and ADI.

- Twenty healthcare utilization models were estimated to predict annualized counts of hospital admissions, hospital days, emergency room visits, outpatient visits for physical or mental health problems, ambulance trips, radiology services, telehealth visits, laboratory services, and various types of prescription pharmaceuticals. These utilization models were estimated using a Poisson regression approach with a log link function. Predictors for these models included the same variables used for the chronic condition models, along with indicators for actually having any of the 23 chronic conditions.

- Sixteen unit-cost regression models for the utilization types mentioned above were estimated assuming a Gamma cost distribution. Age groupings, gender, and indicators for living where ADI scores were either low, medium, or high were also used as predictors for these models[4]. The unit cost predictions were multiplied by the healthcare utilization predictions, to predict total healthcare expenditures per person per year. These were then trended forward to put in year 2022 values, for the initial release of HEAT.

Next, survey data from the US Behavioral Risk Factor Surveillance System (BRFSS) files maintained by the Centers for Disease Control and Prevention [9] were used to estimate the probabilities each person would report having problems related to tobacco use, obesity, nutrition problems, or alcohol use problems. Four logistic regression models (one for each type of problem) were used with survey data from 2016 to 2020 to estimate these probabilities. Multiple years of BRFSS data were used because survey questions about these problems were scattered across years. Descriptions of the survey questions used to measure these outcomes can be found for any of the years on https://www.cdc.gov/brfss/annual_data. Predictors for these logistic models included age, gender, income, metropolitan statistical area of residence, and having one or more diagnosed cancers, arthritis, asthma, stroke, diabetes, kidney disease, or mental health problems.

The chronic condition, utilization, and unit cost models noted above were trained and tested using an 80/20 split of the insurance plan training data set from 2018. The risk factor models were trained and tested using a 70/30 split of the BRFSS training data set from 2016 to 2020.

Appendix 4. Additional variables created for HEAT

Several additional variables were created for HEAT as well. These utilized the predictions and employee census data described above, and other federal data sources to create metrics related to healthcare affordability, residence in primary care or mental health shortage areas, residence in market areas with highly concentrated inpatient facilities, expected time lost from work to receive medical care, employee perceptions

[4] Age groups boundaries were set a 0-5, 5-9, 10-14, 15-19, 20-29, 30-39, 40-49, 50-59, and greater than age 60.

of the adequacy of their health plans, and measures of provider costs and quality in the areas where insured members live.

Healthcare Affordability estimates for 2022 were based on estimated family income, demographics, employee contributions and out-of-pocket payments, plan design information provided by individual clients, and individual's predicted healthcare expenditures for the year. Low Affordability was designated as having expected spending that would exceed 10% of family income in the year. Medium Affordability was designated as having expected spending that would lie between 5 and 10% of family income. High Affordability was designated as having expected spending on healthcare that would be less than 5% of family income.

Mental Health and Primary Care Health Professional Shortage Areas (HPSAs) were defined using criteria from the federal Health Resources and Services Administration. These criteria are available on https://data.hrsa.gov/tools/shortage-area/hpsa-find[1].

HEAT uses zip codes provided in the employee census file to tie residences to counties. Then aggregated county level data processed by HRSA's Rural Health Information Hub as of November 2022 identify counties that are entirely in a HPSA (High risk), partially in a HPSA (Medium risk), or not in a HPSA (Low risk).

Residence in Areas Where Inpatient Services Are Highly Concentrated was defined using data from the Health Care Cost Institute—HCCI [20]. The dataset used for this is on https://healthcostinstitute.org/hcci-originals/hmi-interactive#HMI-Concentration-Index.

The HCCI divides hospital concentrations into four categories, based on its Herfindahl-Hirschman Index—HHI [21], which is a common measure of market concentration. HEAT further aggregates the two most concentrated categories into one, resulting in three categories defined in **Table A1**.

Expected Time Lost from Work was assumed to be 1 day for each day spent as a hospital inpatient and/or for each outpatient/doctor's office visit. This value was capped at an annual maximum of 260 working days per year. The resulting value was then monetized using this formula:

Concentration (HCCI)	Herfindahl–Hirschman Index	Concentration (HEAT)
Unconcentrated	0–1500	Low
Moderately Concentrated	1500 - 2500	Medium
Highly Concentrated	2500 - 4000	High
Very Highly Concentrated	4000 – 10,000	High

Table A1.
Categorizing the Herfindahl-Hirschman Index to Create Provider Concentration Scores.

Category	Cost and Quality Score	Cost Score	Quality Score
Low	0–40	0–40	0–40
Medium	41–60	41–60	41–60
High	61–100	61–100	61–100

Table A2.
Creating cost and quality categories.

$$Timeawaycost = \frac{EmployeeAnnualIncome}{260} \times timeawaydays \qquad (1)$$

Provider Cost and Quality Scores for HEAT were created for doctors and other providers who bill commercial insurance companies for care. These scores were aggregated to the county level by experts at Garner Health. HEAT shows the average Cost and Quality Scores separately and combined for providers located in each county where Employees live. Details for how these scores are calculated for individual doctors and other providers are shown in Garner's methods white paper [22] but a high-level summary is as follows.

- Cost and Quality Score: A relative score between 0 and 100 based on the combination of cost and quality scores associated with each primary care and specialist provider in the county
- Cost Score: A relative score between 0 and 100 based on allowed charges billed by these providers per member per month
- Quality Score: A relative score between 0 and 100 based on sick days (time lost from work) associated with the admissions, visits and procedures used to treat the conditions provided as treatment by each doctor or other provider in the county.

These scores are then categorized as either low, medium, or high, as shown in **Table A2**.

Author details

Ronald J. Ozminkowski[1*], Wendy M. Smith[2], Weiyee Lee[3], Phil Salinger[4], Pedro Jofre Lora[4], Brandon Young[5] and Sandip Gupta[5]

1 Commercial Analytics, Aon plc, Chicago, US

2 World Class Health, New York, US

3 Aon Centre for Innovation and Analytics, Aon plc, Singapore

4 Research and Data Science, Garner Health, New York, US

5 Commercial, Garner Health, New York, US

*Address all correspondence to: ron.ozminkowski@aon.com

References

[1] Aon plc Analytics Based Upon Information Contained in Employer Costs for Employee Compensation. 2023. Available from: https://www.bls.gov/archives/ecec_061623.pdf [Accessed: September 23, 2024]

[2] Commonwealth Fund: State of U.S. Health Insurance in 2022: Findings from the Commonwealth Fund Biennial Health Insurance Survey. Available from: https://www.commonwealthfund.org/publications/isssue-briefs/2022/sep/state-us-health-insurance-2022-biennial-survey [Accessed: July 5, 2024]

[3] Lopes L, Montero A, Presiado M, Hame L. Americans' Challenges with Health Care Costs. Kaiser Family Foundation; 2024. Available from: https://www.kff.org/health-costs/issue-brief/americans-challenges-with-health-care-costs [Accessed: November 5, 2024]

[4] Penchansky R, Thomas JW. The concept of access: Definition and relationship to consumer satisfaction. Medical Care. 1981;**19**:127-140

[5] Ricketts TC, Goldsmith LJ. Access in health services research: The battle of the frameworks. Nursing Outlook. 2005;**53**:274-280

[6] Garner Health. Complications: A Proprietary Analysis of Complications Following Joint Replacement in Greater Dallas Area. Garner Health; 2024

[7] Aon plc. Key Trends in U.S. Benefits for 2024 and Beyond. Available from: https://www.aon.com/en/insights/articles/key-trends-in-us-benefits-for-2024-and-beyond [Accessed: July 5, 2024]

[8] Shiny. Easy Web Applications in R. Available from: https://www.rstudio.com/products/shiny/ [Accessed: July 5, 2024]

[9] Richardson LD, Norris M. Access to health and health care: How race and ethnicity matter. Mount Sinai Journal of Medicine: A Journal of Translational and Personized Medicine. 2010;**77**:166-177. DOI: 10.1002/msj.20174 [Accessed: July 5, 2024]

[10] Prentice JC, Pizer SD. Delayed access to care and mortality. Health Services Research. 2006;**42**(2):644-662. DOI: 10.1111/j.1475-6773.2006.00626x

[11] Asch SM, Kerr EA, Keesey J, et al. Who is at risk for receiving poor-quality health care? New England Journal of Medicine. 2006;**354**:1147-1156

[12] University of Wisconsin-Madison, Population Health Institute. 2020 County Health Rankings. Available from: https://uwphi.pophealth.wisc.edu/wp-content/uploads/sites/316/2020/04/CHR2020_WI_statereport.pdf [Accessed: July 5, 2024]

[13] United States Census. Current Population Survey Tables for Family Income. Available from: https://www.census.gov/data/table/time-series/demo/income-poverty/cps-finc.html [Accessed: July 7, 2024]

[14] Ozminkowski RJ, Metcalfe L. Enhancing enhanced care management. Journal of Occupational and Environmental Medicine. 2024;**6**:e252-e254

[15] Inserro A. Nearly 75% of US Hospital Markets Highly Concentrated, HCCI Report Shows. 2019. Available from: https://www.ajmc.com/. [Accessed: March 8, 2024]

[16] Health Resources and Services Administration (HRSA), Health Professional Shortage Areas. Available from: https://data.hrsa.gov/tools/shortage-area/hpsa-find [Accessed: July 5, 2024]

[17] University of Wisconsin Center for Health Disparities Research, School of Medicine and Public Health. Neighborhood Atlas. Available from: https://www.neighborhoodatlas.medicine.wisc.edu [Accessed: July 5, 2024]

[18] Centers for Disease Control. Behavioral Risk Factor Surveillance System, Annual survey data are Available from: https://www.cdc.gov/brfss/annual_data [Accessed: July 5, 2024]

[19] Databricks SDK for Python. Databricks on AWS. Available from: https://docs.databricks.com/en/dev-tools/sdk-python.html#:~:text:You%20can%20use%20the%20Databricks, Python%20from%20a%20Databricks%20notebook. [Accessed: July 18, 2024]

[20] Health Care Cost Institute—HCCI. Hospital Concentration Index: An Analysis of U.S. Hospital Market Concentration. Available from: https://healthcostinstitute.org/hcci-originals/hmi-interactive#HMI-Concentration-Index [Accessed: July 5, 2024]

[21] U.S. Department of Justice, Antitrust Division. Herfindahl-Hirschman Index. Available from: https://www.justice.gov/atr/herfindahl-hirschman-index [Accessed: July 5, 2024]

[22] Garner Health. A Center for Clinical Excellence in Your Neighborhood.pdf. Available from: https://www.getgarner.com/whitepapers [Accessed: July 5, 2024]

Chapter 3

Perspective Chapter: Developing Skills to Save Lives by Air and by Sea

Luis Alberto Camputaro, Humberto Alcides Urbina Vasquez and Alejandro Jose Duarte Cuellar

Abstract

This document outlines the development and implementation of an integrated medical emergency response system in El Salvador. The system has been scheduled since 2021 and will be put into operation in November 2023. It focuses on air and sea transport capabilities to enhance the efficiency and reach of medical services in critical situations. A robust medical emergency system equipped with ground ambulances, air medical transport *via* helicopters, and maritime transport with rescue boats is essential for timely and effective emergency response. The system aims to ensure rapid stabilization and safe transport of patients to specialized medical facilities, particularly in geographically challenging areas. The enhanced medical emergency system in El Salvador, supported by trained personnel and modern transport methods, significantly improves the nation's capability to respond to emergencies effectively, regardless of geographic challenges. Continuous training and integrating air and sea transport are critical to maintaining a high standard of emergency medical services.

Keywords: emergency medical transport, air medical evacuation, maritime rescue, medical training programs, El Salvador emergency services

1. Introduction

A robust and well-equipped medical emergency system guarantees quick and efficient care in critical situations. It includes many ground ambulances, an aeromedical transport system with several helicopters, and a maritime transport system with boats. It offers multiple benefits that significantly improve emergency response and, ultimately, save lives.

An emergency medical system with a large fleet of ambulances allows rapid response in urban and suburban areas. Ground ambulances are designed to provide immediate medical care and stabilization at the scene and safely transport patients to medical facilities.

The Emergency Medical Service (Servicio de Emergencias Médicas -SEM- in original language) has 140 equipped ambulances, reducing waiting times and ensuring that resources are always available, even during periods of high demand.

The aeromedical transport system has three fully equipped helicopters, adding a vital response layer when critical time or ground access is limited. Helicopters can quickly reach remote or congested locations, providing fast, direct transportation to specialized medical centers. This is especially beneficial in cases of severe trauma, accidents in rural areas, or natural disasters, where every minute counts for the patient's survival.

On the other hand, the maritime transfer system, equipped with three fully equipped boats, is crucial for coastal areas or areas with significant bodies of water, such as our country's. Rescue boats can access places inaccessible by land and provide immediate medical care and safe transportation from ships, islands, or riverside areas. This component is essential for comprehensive coverage, ensuring that emergency medical care is available in all situations and geographies.

A well-equipped medical emergency system with ambulances, helicopters, and boats ensures a rapid, efficient, and versatile response appropriate to each country's geography, drastically improving patients' chances of survival and recovery in emergencies.

2. The medical emergency system (SEM)

The Directorate of the SEM is an institution attached to the Ministry of Health that, through medical and technological resources, provides pre-hospital and emergency care to victims who have suffered injuries or a sudden illness. They can be treated on-site to stabilize and then transfer the patient to the nearest hospital free of charge. The institutional priorities are summarized in national coverage, by land, air, or sea, to provide timely, quality, and warm pre-hospital medical care to the Salvadoran population [1].

The SEM was inaugurated for the Metropolitan area on December 17, 2013. It had a relevant role during the COVID-19 pandemic. Therefore, the Ministry of Health expanded its operational bases to the entire national territory, inaugurating this new phase on November 29, 2023. The medical and nursing teams of the SEM ambulances transferred the patients from their place of detection, transferring the vast majority to the El Salvador Hospital. A 1000-bed hospital was inaugurated by the government of El Salvador on June 20, 2020, to centralize and treat patients affected by the pandemic or, eventually, another neighboring hospital for patients who did not tolerate long-distance transport.

El Salvador is a small country in extension (21,040 km^2), but its geographical characteristics make it difficult to travel long distances, causing delays. During the rainy season, the roads can also be affected.

The Government of El Salvador, through its Ministry of Health, is reshaping the National Health System post-pandemic, increasing and strengthening the experience acquired during it.

Investment in medical equipment and specialized human resource training has increased; in this sense, investment is being made in strengthening the response of medical emergency systems.

The SEM, strengthened by the COVID-19 experience, continues to provide response, stabilization, and transfer services, both in accident events and in obstetric and neonatal emergencies, to the elderly and the general population at the national level that requires its assistance.

Implementing this updated and agile system requires continuous staff training, accompanied by the design and application of relevant response protocols that allow an integrated emergency response; therefore, specialized training of health personnel in procedural and logistical aspects is increasingly necessary.

The Solidarity Fund for Health (FOSALUD in original language) [2] and the SEM are the main actors in medical emergencies in any territory of the country.

Both institutions requested the Specialized Institute "Hospital El Salvador" (IEHES in original language) for Academic and Logistical support in designing and delivering short training courses in air and maritime transfer.

The new medical emergency system has been operating since November 2023 with its fleet of ambulances, three helicopters, and three ambulance boats, with a staff of 157 doctors, 286 emergency teleoperators, and 146 medical assistants.

The objective is to continue the optimization of the response in the "golden hours" originally described by Dr. R. Adams Cowley [3] in the different pathologies.

3. Geography of El Salvador

El Salvador is in Central America and is the only country that does not have a border with the Caribbean Sea [4]. It is the most densely populated in the region, with 6.4 million inhabitants. It borders to the south with the North Pacific Ocean, the northwest with Guatemala, and the north and northeast with Honduras. In the southeast, the Gulf of Fonseca separates it from Nicaragua. El Salvador is about the same size as Slovenia or Israel but has the population size of Libya and Lebanon.

It is a territory of volcanic origin with a tropical climate. Although the central plateau makes up only 25% of the area, it contains most of the population and the country's most populated cities. This plain is 50 km wide and has an average elevation of 600 m above sea level. The terrain is undulating, with some escarpments, lava fields, and geysers.

Its geography also has around 300 rivers. The most important is the Lempa River, which originates in Guatemala, crosses the Sierra Madre, flows through the central plateau, and crosses the volcanic chain to empty into the Pacific. It is the only navigable river. The other rivers are short and drain through the lowlands or flow from the central plateau, forming gorges in the volcanic chain on the way to the Pacific.

In the interior highlands, there are numerous lakes of volcanic origin. Many are surrounded by mountains that have steep slopes. The largest is Lake Ilopango, at 440 m and 72 km^2, east of the capital. Other lakes are Lake Coatepeque, at 746 m and 26 km^2, to the west, and Lake Güija, on the border with Guatemala, at 430 mm and 45 km^2.

This geography requires a strengthened medical emergency system with the capacity to carry out safe and agile transfers of highly complex patients and avoid delays caused by geographical conditions.

Risk assessments were carried out to ensure efficiency in emergency transfers, and gaps in the need for rapid emergency response appropriate to our territory were identified.

The team was used to program requirements in the WHO Air Transport Manual and the International Civil Aviation Organization (ICAO) standards for search and rescue (SAR) services. In addition, the IAMSAR guidelines, developed jointly with the International Maritime Organization (IMO), provide detailed guidelines for aviation SAR operations, including the need for supplies and personnel adequately trained and certified according to international standards.

4. First phase

4.1 Air transfer

4.1.1 Needs diagnosis

Rapidly detecting severe illnesses and accidents, whether in traffic or sports, is crucial for stabilizing the patient and their evacuation to a specialized center. However, highly trained transfer experts must take these actions to achieve effective care. This implies that these professionals must possess skills beyond simple risk classification and damage control to guarantee that the patient arrives at the place of specialized care in the best possible conditions.

In this sense, air transport with trained personnel is a very beneficial option for severely compromised patients located a considerable distance outside the metropolitan area of San Salvador [5]. This is because travel time is significantly reduced, which improves the possibility of adequate care in a specialized reference center. Additionally, specialized care during the "therapeutic window" has proven to be especially effective for seriously ill patients or accident victims.

It is essential to understand that the training and skills of the personnel in charge of the transfer are vital in guaranteeing the safety and effectiveness of this process. Therefore, it is essential that the professionals in charge of air transport are adequately trained to deal with emergencies and can carry out the necessary procedures to ensure safe and effective evacuation of patients.

4.1.2 Course objective, target population, and graduation profile

The training of personnel responsible for the safe transfer of patients in emergencies for the provision of specialized care was strengthened, and technical-administrative tools were provided for the analysis and evaluation of response mechanisms.

It was carried out by doctors and nurses selected from the medical emergency system (SEM) and emergency medicine resident doctors from the Rosales National Hospital. This highly complex hospital receives the most seriously ill patients since it has all the specialties.

During the course taught by aero-evacuation experts, the students were encouraged to acquire and strengthen skills that allow them autonomy to participate in the patient's classification, stabilization, and transfer under life support for a safe transfer by air. This will minimize the risk of complications after the transfer and maintain safety standards for the user and the healthcare team.

Emergency medicine residents from the Rosales National Hospital, San Rafael National Hospital, and Zacamil National Hospital were invited to this training.

To develop professional skills in the different techniques and procedures necessary for the identification and control of risk, management of emergencies, preparation,

	Modules
1	Aero medical evacuation, history, and development
2	Atmosphere and physiology of flight
3	Aeromedical evacuation standards and procedures
4	Aeromedical evacuation in pediatrics and neonatology
5	Aero medical evacuation of obstetric patient
6	Aeromedical evacuation in polytraumatized patients
7	Evacuation in special situations
8	Aeromedical evacuation in the military field
9	Practical integration workshop

Table 1.
Aeromedical transfer course program.

and equipment of the aircraft that allow safe and effective air transport, nine modules were designed, the design specific for this training activity with a duration of 4 months (**Table 1**).

4.1.3 Teaching-learning methodology

The IEHES strategy generates knowledge construction from practice, allowing students to acquire experiential experience and "know-how" skills.

To acquire sufficient experiential experience, the course was conducted in person, in two commissions, to maintain an optimal teacher-student relationship. The course was taught entirely at the Ilopango Airport, where the air base of the three fully equipped medical helicopters is located on the integrated health system.

The theoretical knowledge acquired in the different modules was evaluated upon completion through an online exam with a multiple-choice question strategy, which had to be answered in at most 1 hour on the indicated day. The pilots are being evaluated through field workshops at Ilopango airport.

The final exam consisted of a multiple-accident simulation.

It was designed with teaching staff and ship crews; the students did not know the simulation script. To affirm the realism of the simulations, nursing students participated as "patients" adequately made up (**Figures 1–6**).

4.1.4 Results

Seventy-five students participated: doctors, nurses, and emergency medicine residents.

Sixty-two passed the intermediate exams and workshops that enabled them to take the final Multiple Casualty Simulation exams, of which 52 passed the University Aero Medical Evacuation Course.

The approved students became part of the helicopter crew in charge of aeromedical transfer or recipients of transfer at Rosales National Hospital.

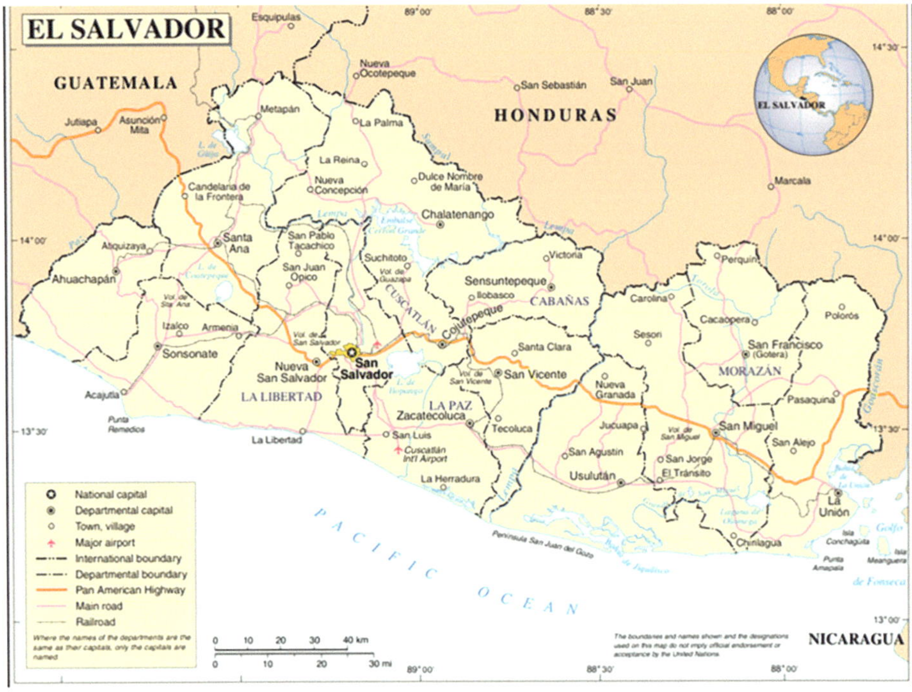

Figure 1.
Map of the Republic of El Salvador.

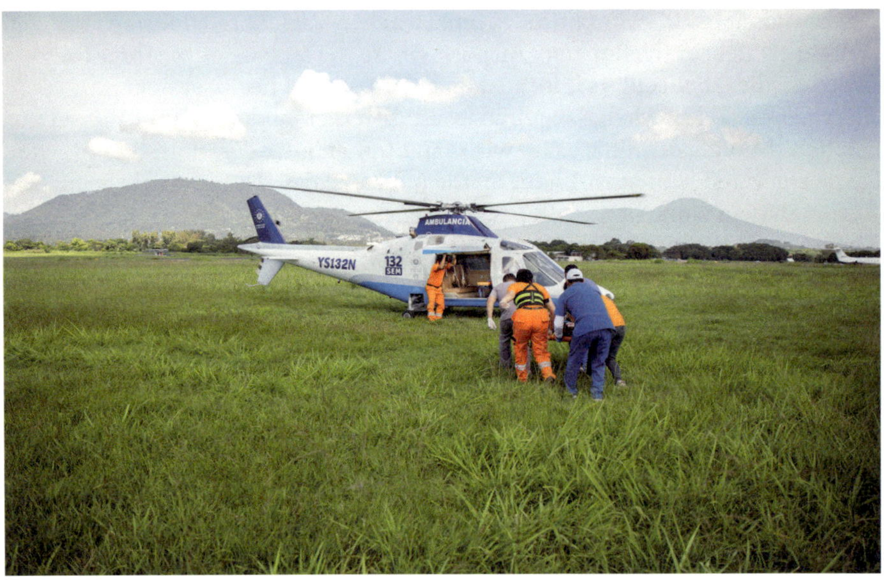

Figure 2.
Ilopango Airport air base.

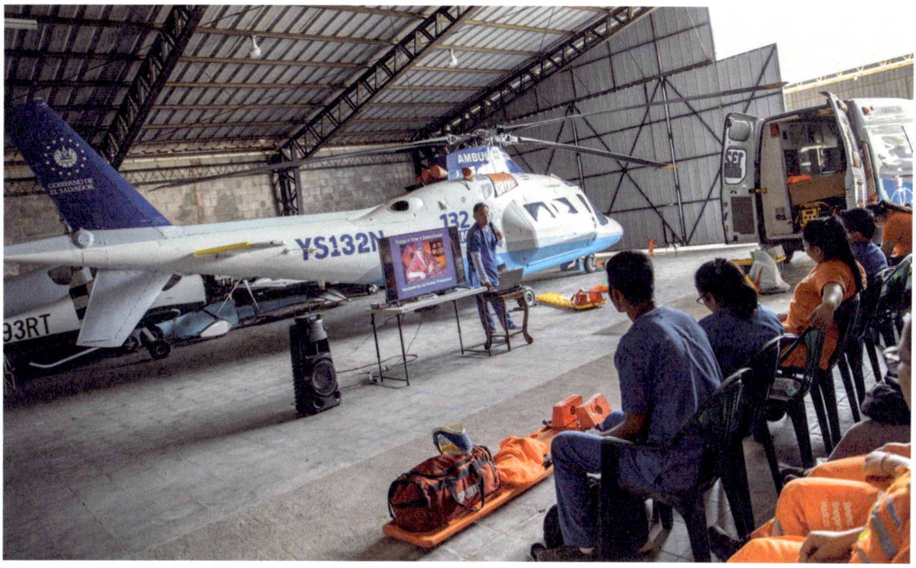

Figure 3.
Theoretical classes in hangar.

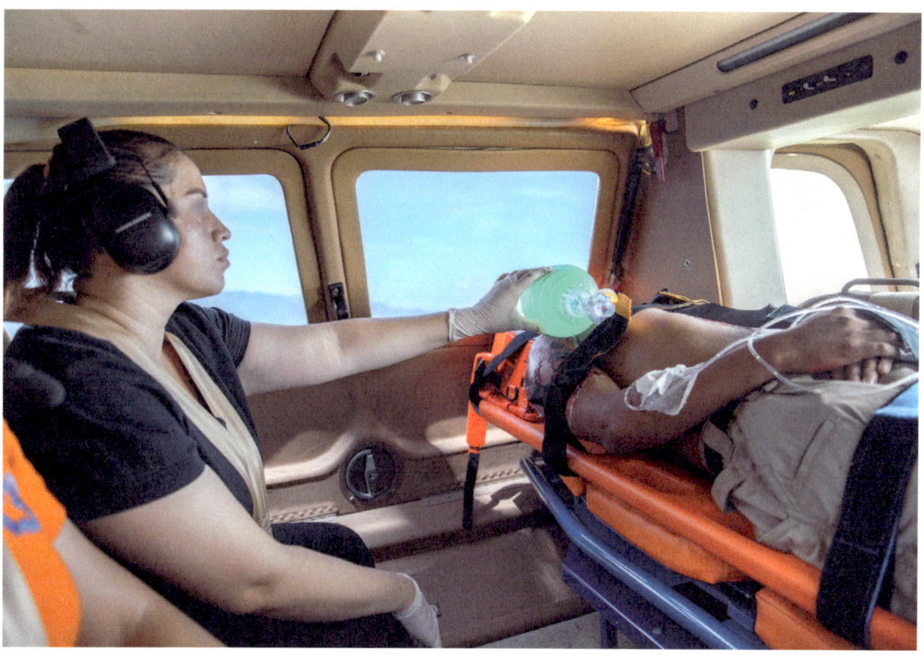

Figure 4.
Students practicing patient transfer on mechanical ventilatory assistance.

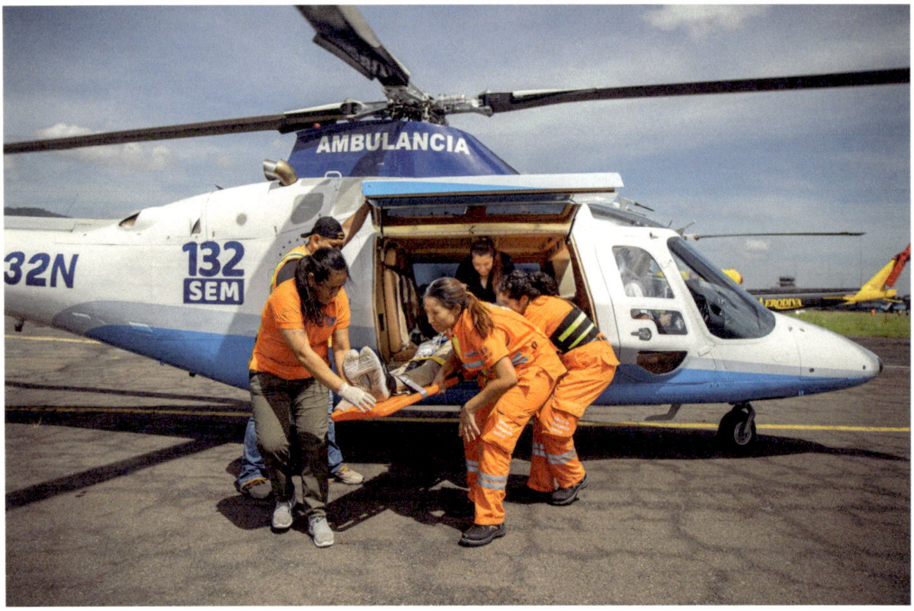

Figure 5.
Students practicing boarding and landing critically ill patient.

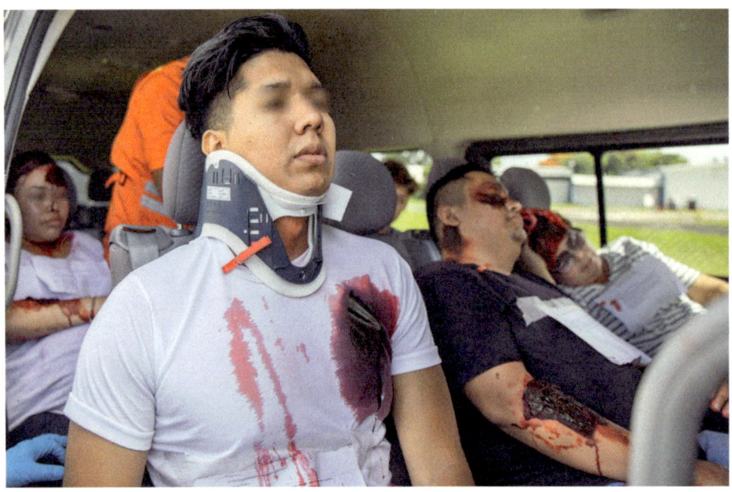

Figure 6.
Final evaluation workshop. Simulation with the collaboration of nursing school students. Make-up and scripts according to the role to be developed.

5. Second stage

5.1 Sea transfer

5.1.1 Needs diagnosis

Implementing the advanced sea-air transfer course for serious patients is a pressing need in remote coastal areas and islands. This imperative need arises because of

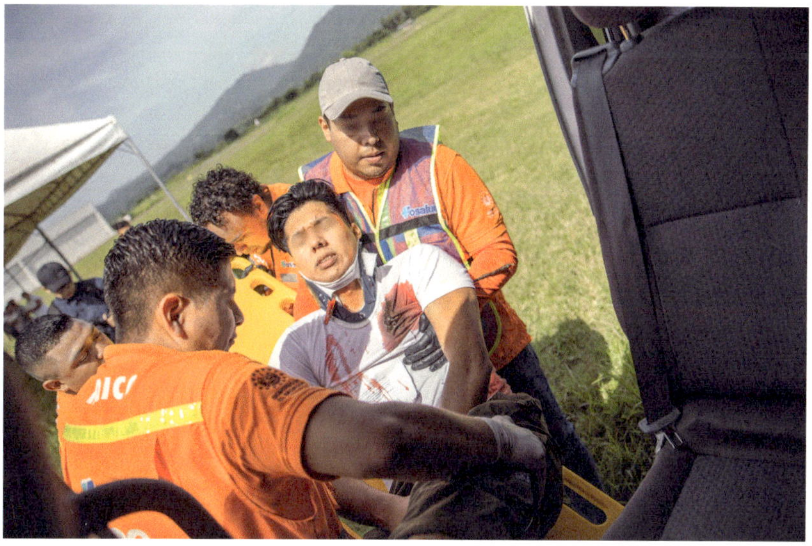

Figure 7.
Nursing school collaborators in the evaluation workshop, key personnel for evaluating competencies.

the exceptional circumstances that surround the medical care of patients who require highly complex care, to which are added the victims of drowning in these geographically isolated regions (**Figure** 7).

Remote geography and limited access to emergency medical services must be addressed. Urgently transferring patients from remote locations to reference hospitals becomes a complex task that requires specialized training to ensure the safety and well-being of the patient.

Beyond seriously ill patients who require transfer, the new conditions as a country have significantly increased the attraction of residents and tourists to aquatic activities, increasing the risks of aquatic accidents, including drowning. Consequently, creating a specialized diploma in maritime transfer linked to air transfer is a priority to equip health personnel in these areas with the necessary skills and knowledge to face these situations effectively.

5.1.2 Course objective, target population, and graduation profile

Contribute to training personnel responsible for transferring patients in emergencies to provide specialized, safe, and autonomous care aimed at users of the emergency system's services, providing technical-administrative tools for analyzing and evaluating response mechanisms.

The medical personnel of the health units in the Islas area attended the course. This course offered places to applicants from other civil or military health professions in charge of the maritime transport of patients to general or specialized hospitals as appropriate who also met the psychological, physical, and skill requirements regulated by the medical emergency system.

The IEHES, within its principles, considers that training should reach the student and not vice versa, which is why this course had a hybrid format. Synchronous online classes during weekdays, recording in the virtual classroom enabled for this purpose, with the objective that students who could not be synchronous did not miss classes.

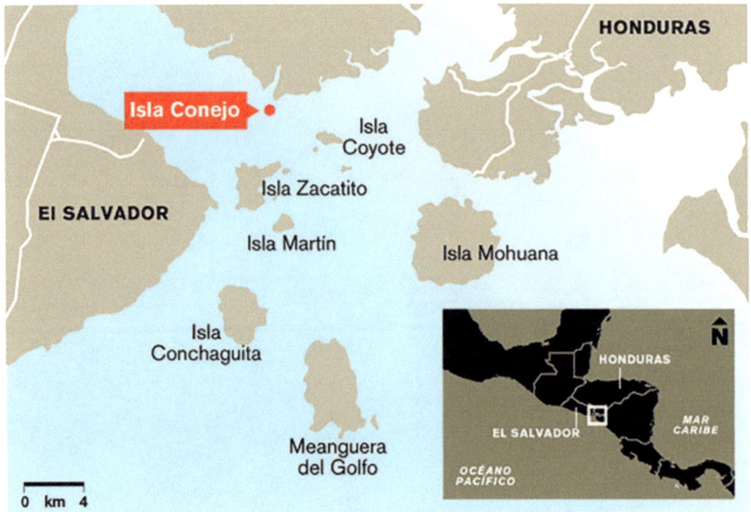

Figure 8.
Islands zone. Republic of El Salvador.

Due to the distances and availability of local participants' mobilization, in-person workshops are held in the field every 15 days in two commissions: Zona la Unión and Zona Costa del Sol (**Figure 8**).

The students were strengthened by acquiring the skills that would allow them to autonomously carry out triage, leading the preparation and coordination of the patient for a safe transfer by sea with one of the three fully equipped medical boats. If necessary, the student could continue by air to another highly complex hospital.

Like the Aeromedical Transfer Course, exams were taken at the end of each module and must be completed on the indicated day and time.

The qualified students took the final exam, which again consisted of a simulation of multiple victims in an Island scenario. The School of Nursing supported the final evaluation by providing us with the "victims" suitably made up. Also, the students had no knowledge of the simulation script in this simulation.

The course developed 8 modules that lasted for 3 months (**Table 2**).

	Modules
1	Intervention in Aquatic Care - Communication System (CCSEM).
2	Pathophysiology of Drowning-Diving.
3	Rescue and Initial Evaluation - Vital Signs.
4	Basic, Advanced and Trauma Life Support.
5	Stabilization and Preparation for Critical Transfer.
6	Safe Patient Transfer- SRRE- SRRI.
7	Considerations in Pediatrics and Pregnancy
8	Final Drill of Multiple Victim Incidents (35 victims) Land – Maritime Air Integrator (Simultaneous Islands).

Table 2.
Maritime air transfer modules program.

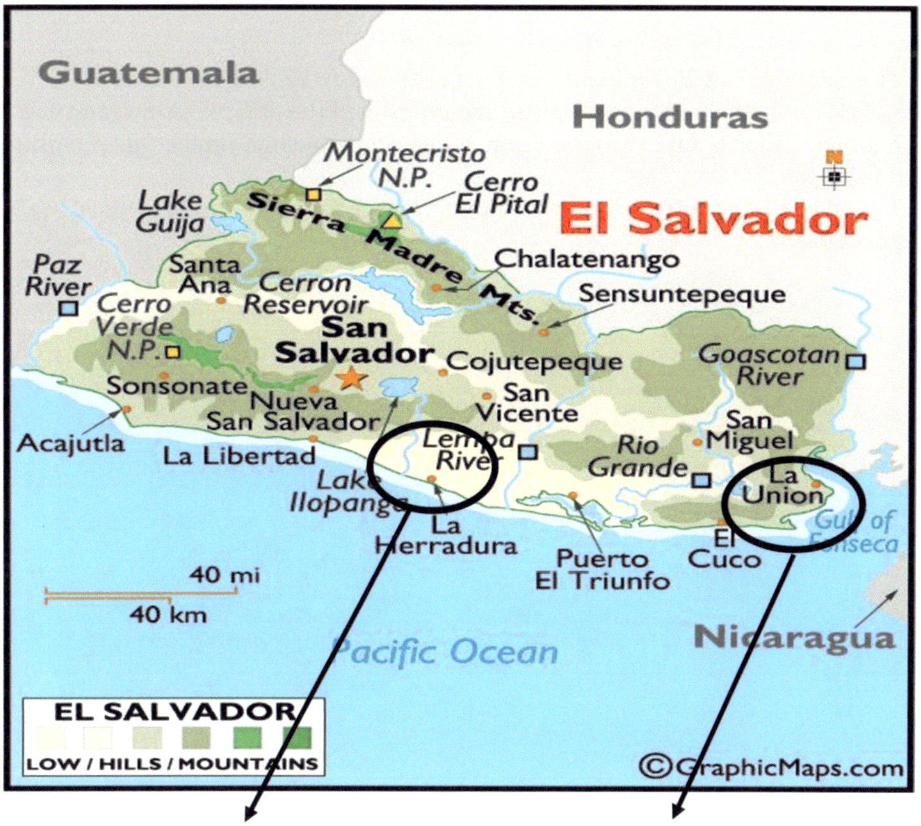

Figure 9.
Location of the field practices of the La Unión Commission, Costa del Sol Commission.

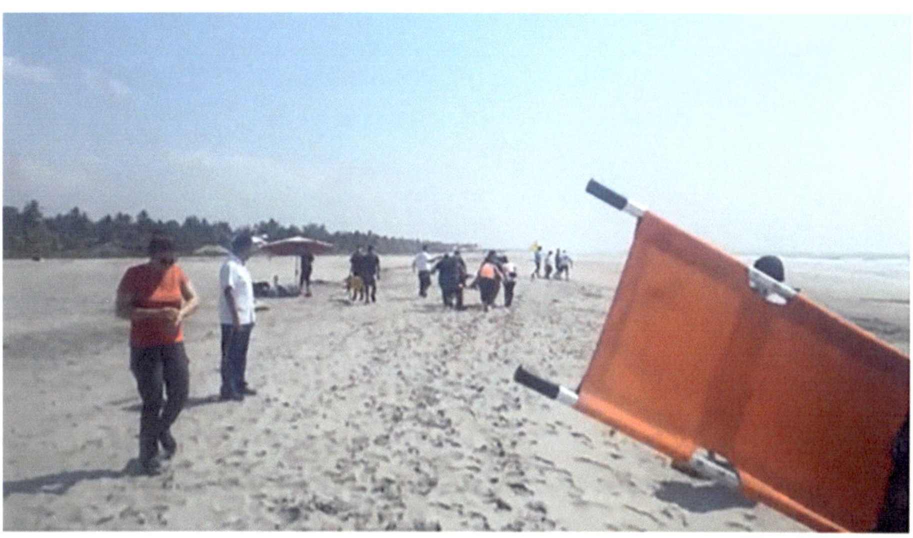

Figure 10.
Students in a real maritime rescue scenario.

5.1.3 Results

This program had 200 students, of whom 120 met the 80% connection to the virtual classes (synchronous or asynchronous), passed the module exams, and was therefore qualified to take the final exam, which consisted of a simulation of multiple victims on the island of Tasajera.

A total of 82 students passed, who became part of the crews of the medical boats (**Figures 9–15**).

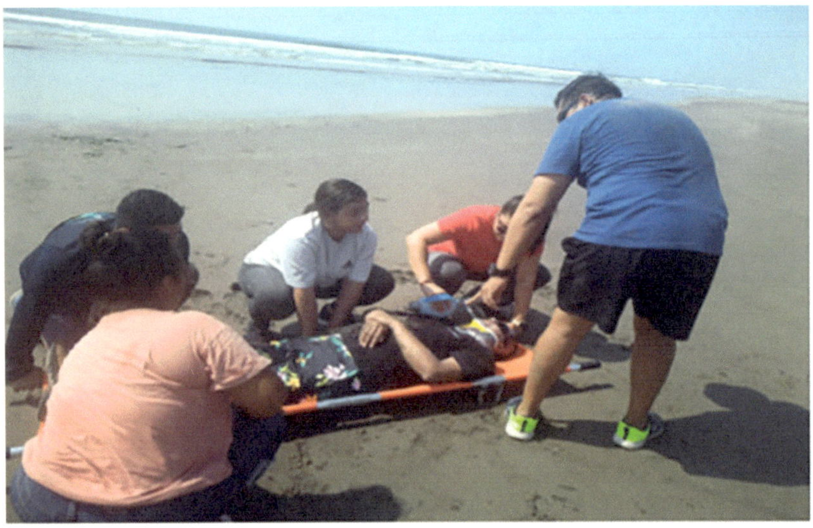

Figure 11.
Students practicing resuscitation and transfer of critically ill patient in beach setting.

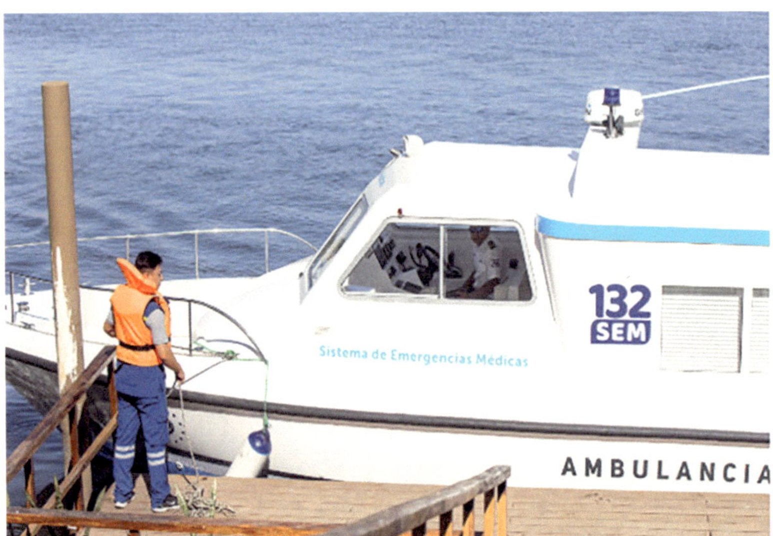

Figure 12.
Final evaluation workshop on maritime transfer, with the participation of the ambulance boats of the medical emergency system.

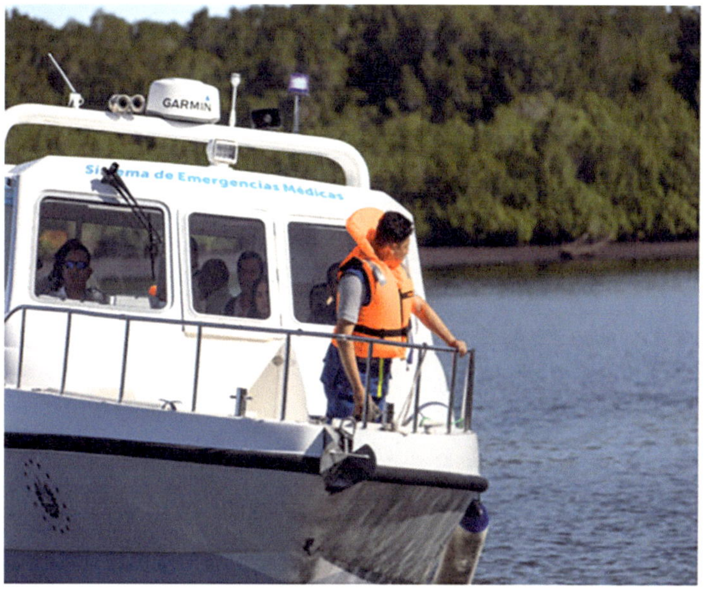

Figure 13.
The final evaluation workshop for the ambulance boat crew had the logistical collaboration of the Naval Base of La Unión.

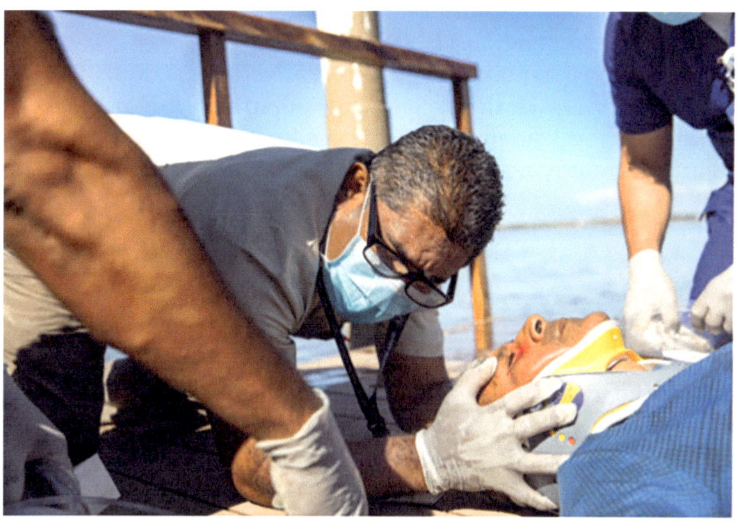

Figure 14.
Simulation of resuscitation and stabilization of a patient with multiple trauma due to a maritime accident.

6. Comments and discussion

The "Saving Lives by Air and Sea" initiative in El Salvador represents a significant step toward enhancing the country's emergency medical services (EMS). This initiative, structured in phases to address aerial and maritime emergency responses, underscores the need for specialized training and equipment to meet El Salvador's unique geographical challenges.

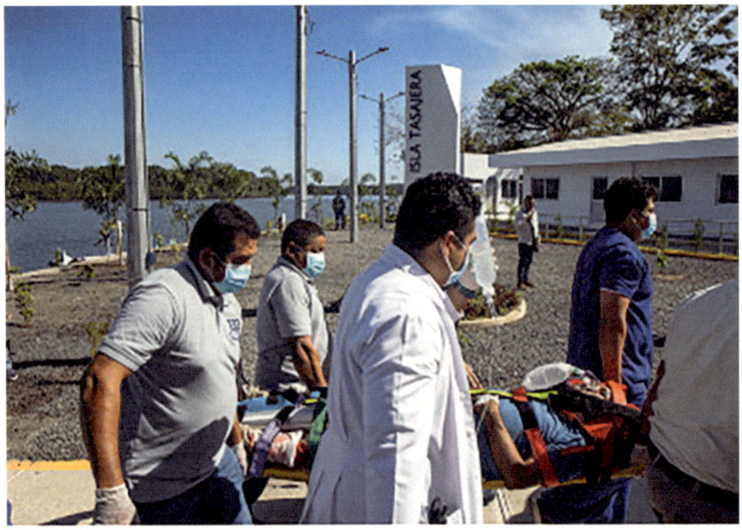

Figure 15.
Simulation. Arrival of a stabilized patient at the Tasajera Island Emergency Care Center (CAE).

6.1 Experiences with air and sea transport in Central America

In general, the countries of Central America have limited but growing capacities for medical transfers by air and, to a lesser extent, by sea.

Geography and infrastructure are key factors affecting the availability and efficiency of these services. Health systems depend, to a greater or lesser extent, on cooperation between government agencies, armed forces, and relief organizations, which is essential to improving response capabilities in medical emergencies.

6.1.1 Guatemala

Guatemala has a 122-emergency system, managed by the Volunteer Firefighters, Municipal Firefighters, and the Red Cross. There is capacity for air transfers, especially in rural areas where access by road transport is limited. The Guatemalan Air Force is also involved in medical evacuations. The use of sea transport is limited and is concentrated in coastal and lake areas.

6.1.2 Honduras

In Honduras, Permanent Commission on Contingencies (COPECO) and other rescue organizations have air evacuation capabilities, especially in natural disasters. The Honduran Air Force plays a crucial role in these transfers. Sea transfers are more common in Honduras, the Mosquitia region, and the Bay Islands, where resources are more accessible.

6.1.3 Nicaragua

Nicaragua has an emergency system includes the General Fire Department and the Nicaraguan Red Cross. The Nicaraguan Air Force can also provide emergency services. However, the infrastructure for maritime transport is limited and is mainly used on the Caribbean Coast.

6.1.4 Costa Rica

Costa Rica has a well-developed emergency system, with 911 as the central number. The Emergency Service Air Surveillance of the Ministry of Public Security carries out emergency air transports. In addition, the Costa Rican Red Cross has agreements with private companies to use helicopters. As for maritime transport, the Red Cross and the National Coast Guard Service are actively involved, especially in tourist and coastal areas.

6.1.5 Panama

Panama's emergency system is managed by the National Civil Protection System (SINAPROC) and the National Aeronaval Service (SENAN), which has air and maritime capabilities. SENAN carries out medical evacuations in hard-to-reach areas and coastal zones.

6.2 Strengthening EMS capabilities

Historically, the healthcare system in El Salvador has faced challenges in providing timely and high-quality emergency medical services (EMS) due to the lack of certified resources for managing aerial and maritime emergencies. However, substantial efforts have been made to overcome these limitations. Our system has consistently aimed to offer prompt and quality medical care in critical out-of-hospital emergencies. The primary goal has always been to stabilize patients at the scene, prepare them for transport, and ultimately save lives while minimizing the risk of long-term complications.

The initiative's first phase, focused on aerial transport, highlights the critical role of rapid response in medical emergencies. The integration of helicopters into the EMS framework addresses the limitations of terrestrial transport, particularly in remote or congested areas. This is crucial given El Salvador's varied topography, which includes volcanic terrain, numerous rivers, and dense urban centers. Completing a four-month intensive training program by 52 medical professionals signifies a substantial improvement in the country's ability to provide timely and efficient medical evacuations. These professionals are now equipped to handle severe trauma cases and other critical conditions, ensuring patients receive specialized care within the vital therapeutic window.

6.3 Maritime emergency response

The second phase, emphasizing maritime emergency responses, is equally important. The coastal and insular regions of El Salvador, prone to incidents like drownings and other water-related emergencies, necessitate a robust maritime EMS. The specialized training provided to 82 professionals in this phase ensures that these areas are addressed. The hybrid training model, combining online theoretical classes with practical fieldwork, is particularly effective in accommodating the logistical challenges of training personnel from remote locations.

6.4 Comprehensive emergency coverage

The initiative ensures comprehensive emergency coverage nationwide by equipping the EMS with aerial and maritime capabilities. The deployment of three helicopters and three fully equipped rescue boats provides a multi-faceted approach to emergency response, capable of addressing incidents in various environments. This integrated system improves response times and enhances the overall quality of pre-hospital care, thereby increasing survival rates and reducing long-term complications for patients.

6.5 Challenges and future directions

Despite these advancements, several challenges remain. The sustainability of this enhanced EMS depends on continuous investment in training, equipment maintenance, and system upgrades. Developing standardized protocols and continuous professional development is essential to ensure personnel can handle evolving medical emergencies. Given the high-stress nature of their work, the initiative also needs to consider the psychological and physical well-being of the EMS personnel.

6.6 Impact on public health

The broader impact of this initiative on public health in El Salvador cannot be overstated. By reducing response times and improving the quality of emergency care, the initiative is poised to significantly lower mortality and morbidity rates associated with emergencies. This, in turn, will contribute to a more resilient healthcare system capable of better managing routine emergencies and large-scale disasters, as evidenced by the experience during the COVID-19 pandemic.

6.7 Community involvement and awareness

Another critical aspect of the initiative is community involvement and awareness. Educating the public about the EMS's capabilities and how to utilize these services effectively can enhance the system's overall efficacy. Community-based training programs on basic first aid and emergency response can further augment the EMS's professional services, creating a more robust and responsive emergency care network.

7. Conclusion

In conclusion, the "Saving Lives by Air and Sea" initiative is a transformative project that addresses the urgent need for a versatile and efficient EMS in El Salvador. The successful implementation of aerial and maritime emergency response systems, coupled with the comprehensive training of EMS personnel, sets a new standard for emergency medical care in the region. Continued support and development of this initiative will ensure that it remains a cornerstone of El Salvador's healthcare system, ultimately saving countless lives and improving health outcomes nationwide.

The Specialized Institute "Hospital El Salvador" (IEHES) involvement and commitment have been pivotal in coordinating and executing these competency-based courses. Their dedication has ensured that participants demonstrating the required competencies are certified, reinforcing the country's capacity to handle aerial and maritime emergencies effectively. This initiative, supported by the expertise of teaching specialists and a blended learning approach combining telemedicine for theoretical knowledge and practical skills development, culminates in validated simulations of emergency management, further ensuring the readiness and certification of our emergency responders.

Acknowledgements

We want to extend our heartfelt gratitude to the SEM staff, FOSALUD, students, helicopter crews, and ambulance boat teams for their unwavering commitment and dedication to this program. Your efforts and passion are truly inspiring. We also want to thank the Ministry of Health for their invaluable support, which has been crucial in making this initiative successful.

The development of the program and this paper does not include grants.

Conflict of interest

The authors declare that they have no conflicts of interest.

Notes/thanks/other declarations

These programs are part of the Government's new strategy for transforming the integrated health system, which it strongly supports. The aim is to enhance healthcare delivery and ensure that quality medical services are accessible to everyone. Through the commitment and collaboration of various stakeholders, we are working toward a more efficient and effective healthcare system that meets the needs of our communities.

Acronyms and abbreviations

SEM	Servicio de Emergencias Medicas. Medical Emergency Service
FOSALUD	Fondo Solidario para la Salud. Solidarity Fund for Health
IEHES	Isntituto Especilizado "Hospital El Salvador". Specialized Institute "Hospital El Salvador"

Author details

Luis Alberto Camputaro[1*], Humberto Alcides Urbina Vasquez[2]
and Alejandro Jose Duarte Cuellar[3]

1 Specialized Institute "Hospital El Salvador", San Salvador, El Salvador,
Central America

2 The Solidarity Fund for Health San Salvador, El Salvador, Central America

3 Expert Government of El Salvador, Health Policy, University Institute
IEHES, Global Health, Pandemic Fund, WHO PAHO, and GAVI/COVAX,
San Salvador, El Salvador, Central America

*Address all correspondence to: luis.camputaro@salud.gob.sv

References

[1] Transparency portal. Goberment of El Salvador. El Salvador: Ministry of Health. MINSAL [Internet]. 2024 [Consulted 2024 August]

[2] Transparency portal. Government of El Salvador. El Salvador: Solidarity fund for health. FOSALUD [Internet]. 2024. [Consulted August 2024]

[3] Cowley A, Durham M, Aldred D, et al. Presence of a pre-hospital enhanced care team reduces on scene time and improves triage compliance for stab trauma. Scandinavian Journal of Trauma, Resuscitation and Emergency Medicine. 2019;**27**:86. DOI: 10.1186/s13049-019-0661-z

[4] Republic of El Salvador. Information, geography, culture. Available from: http://republicadeelsalvador.com

[5] Parrino C, Galvagno SM. Aeromedical transport for critically ill patients. Critical Care Clinics. 2024;**40**:481-495

Section 2

International Experiences

Chapter 4

Improving Vaccination Coverage through Access to Vaccination Services in Community Pharmacies: A Case Study of Nigeria's Situation

Yejide Olukemi Oseni

Abstract

Vaccination as a health intervention is one of the most successful and cost-effective methods of addressing preventable disease. Community pharmacies are easily accessible and cost-effective healthcare facilities placed to help improve the capacity and effectiveness of healthcare services. Globally, the use of community pharmacies to deliver vaccination services has been hampered by several factors and policies that do not support pharmacists' participation. With the advent of the COVID-19 pandemic, many developed countries have included community pharmacists and pharmacies in vaccination services to improve coverage. However, challenges still occur in many developing countries. This paper assessed the perception of community pharmacists, perceived benefits, and potential barriers to vaccination services to take up this extended role. It described the delivery of vaccination services in community pharmacies, how their involvement impacted vaccination coverage, and how this experience can be used to support policy revisions in recognizing community pharmacists in vaccination delivery.

Keywords: vaccination services, community pharmacies, community pharmacists, vaccinators, policy review

1. Introduction

Vaccination remains a cornerstone of public health, playing a crucial role in preventing infectious diseases and reducing morbidity and mortality worldwide [1]. However, achieving high vaccination coverage continues to be a significant challenge in many low- and middle-income countries, including Nigeria [2, 3]. The barriers to optimal vaccination coverage in Nigeria are multifaceted, encompassing issues such as inadequate healthcare infrastructure, vaccine supply chain challenges, and widespread misinformation about vaccines [4].

Community pharmacies, with their widespread presence and accessibility, present a promising yet underutilized avenue for enhancing vaccination coverage [5]. Unlike traditional healthcare settings, community pharmacies are often located closer to the population, operate with extended hours, and have established trust within the communities they serve [6, 7]. These attributes position community pharmacies as pivotal players in public health initiatives, particularly in increasing the accessibility of vaccination services [8].

This chapter aims to explore the potential of community pharmacies in Nigeria to improve vaccination coverage. By leveraging the experiences gained during the COVID-19 pandemic, where community pharmacies played a critical role in vaccination efforts [9], this chapter seeks to illustrate how these pharmacies can be integrated into the broader immunization framework. The COVID-19 experience in Nigeria highlighted the ability of community pharmacies to rapidly mobilize resources, reach underserved populations, and effectively administer vaccines [10].

This chapter examines the delivery of vaccination services in community pharmacies through a mixed-methods approach, combining quantitative data from surveys and qualitative insights from interviews. It assesses the improvements in vaccination coverage with the involvement of community pharmacies and discusses how these findings can inform policy reviews that would recognize and formalize the role of community pharmacists (CPs) in immunization service delivery in Nigeria.

Ultimately, this chapter advocates for a policy shift that acknowledges the critical role community pharmacies can play in public health. By integrating community pharmacies into the national immunization strategy, Nigeria can make significant strides in improving vaccination coverage, thereby enhancing overall public health outcomes.

1.1 Context and background

1.1.1 Overview of the healthcare system in Nigeria

Nigeria's healthcare system is characterized by a complex interplay of public and private sectors, with the public sector being the primary provider of healthcare services. The system is structured into primary, secondary, and tertiary levels of care, with primary healthcare being the first point of contact for individuals [11, 12]. The Nigerian government has established numerous healthcare facilities, including primary health centers (PHCs), general hospitals, and teaching hospitals, to cater to the diverse needs of its population [13]. Despite these efforts, the healthcare system faces significant challenges, including inadequate infrastructure, insufficient funding, and a shortage of skilled healthcare professionals [14].

The Nigerian healthcare system is further complicated by geographical disparities, with rural areas often experiencing limited access to healthcare services compared to urban centers [15]. This inequity contributes to the overall difficulty in achieving comprehensive healthcare coverage, including vaccination services [16]. Additionally, Nigeria's healthcare system is burdened by a high disease burden, with prevalent issues such as infectious diseases, maternal and child health concerns, and noncommunicable diseases, all of which place a strain on available resources [17, 18].

1.1.2 Current vaccination strategies and challenges

Nigeria's vaccination strategy involves a combination of routine immunization programs and supplementary immunization activities (SIAs). The National Primary Health Care Development Agency (NPHCDA) oversees these efforts, working to ensure that vaccines are available and administered according to established schedules [19]. Routine immunization focuses on providing vaccines against diseases such as measles, polio, tuberculosis, and Hepatitis B, while SIAs are employed to address specific outbreaks or high-risk areas [20–22].

Despite these strategies, several challenges hinder the effectiveness of vaccination efforts in Nigeria. These challenges include:

1. *Inadequate vaccine supply and distribution*: The vaccine supply chain in Nigeria faces numerous issues, including stockouts, delays in delivery, and inadequate cold chain infrastructure. These problems result in frequent disruptions to vaccination services, impacting coverage rates [23].

2. *Healthcare workforce shortages*: There is a shortage of trained healthcare workers, which affects the delivery of immunization services. This shortage is exacerbated by uneven distribution, with many healthcare workers concentrated in urban areas, leaving rural populations underserved [24].

3. *Public awareness and hesitancy*: Vaccine hesitancy, driven by misinformation and lack of awareness, remains a significant barrier to vaccination coverage. Educational campaigns are often needed to address concerns and misinformation about vaccines [25].

4. *Geographic and economic barriers*: Access to vaccination services is limited in remote and economically disadvantaged areas, where transportation and financial constraints further impede vaccination efforts [26].

1.1.3 Role of community pharmacies in other countries

Community pharmacies have demonstrated considerable potential in enhancing vaccination coverage in various countries around the world. In many high-income countries, community pharmacies have been successfully integrated into national immunization programs, offering a range of vaccines, including seasonal influenza, travel vaccines, and routine childhood immunizations [7, 8]. Benefits of involving community pharmacies in vaccination services include:

1. *Increased accessibility*: Community pharmacies are often more accessible than traditional healthcare facilities, with extended hours and convenient locations. This accessibility allows for higher vaccination uptake, particularly in underserved areas [27].

2. *Convenience and efficiency*: Pharmacies can provide vaccinations with minimal wait times and without the need for prior appointments, which enhances convenience for patients. Additionally, pharmacy staff are trained to manage and administer vaccines efficiently [5, 28].

3. *Integration into health systems*: In countries such as the United States, Canada, and the United Kingdom, community pharmacies are integrated into public health strategies, with protocols in place for vaccine storage, administration, and reporting. This integration has proven effective in increasing vaccination coverage rates [8, 29].

4. *Public trust and education*: Pharmacists are trusted healthcare professionals who play a crucial role in educating patients about vaccines and addressing concerns. Their involvement in vaccination programs helps build public confidence and reduce vaccine hesitancy [9].

Incorporating community pharmacies into Nigeria's vaccination strategy could address several existing challenges by leveraging their accessibility and trusted presence in local communities. This approach has the potential to significantly improve vaccination coverage and overall public health outcomes in Nigeria [30].

2. Research design and methodology

2.1 Research objectives and questions

The primary aim of this study is to enhance vaccination coverage through community pharmacies in Nigeria, leveraging insights from the COVID-19 pandemic as a case study. The specific objectives of the study are as follows:

1. *Assess vaccination services:* Evaluate the current state of vaccination services provided by community pharmacies in Lagos and Oyo States, identifying challenges and gaps.

2. *Examine impact:* Analyze how community pharmacies contributed to vaccination coverage during the COVID-19 pandemic.

3. *Advocate for policy change:* Explore how the findings from the COVID-19 pandemic can be used to advocate for policy changes to formally recognize community pharmacists in vaccination services.

The guiding research questions are as follows:

1. What is the current state of vaccination services provided by community pharmacies in Lagos and Oyo States?

2. How did community pharmacies influence vaccination coverage during the COVID-19 pandemic?

3. What policy recommendations can be made based on the COVID-19 experience to enhance the role of community pharmacists in vaccination services?

2.1.1 Mixed-methods approach

The study adopted a mixed-methods approach, integrating both quantitative and qualitative research to provide a comprehensive evaluation of community pharmacy vaccination services.

2.1.1.1 Quantitative methodology

1. *Study design:* A descriptive cross-sectional survey was employed to assess perceptions, benefits, and barriers related to vaccination services in community pharmacies.

2. *Study participants:* The study participants comprised licensed community pharmacists working in registered community pharmacies located in Lagos and Oyo States, Nigeria. Only those community pharmacies registered with the Pharmacy Council of Nigeria (PCN) and pharmacists who held a valid license with the PCN were included in the study [31]. Exclusion criteria involved non-registered community pharmacies, pharmacists not holding a valid PCN license, as well as all locum, intern, and serving pharmacists.

3. *Sample size and sampling strategy:* Using the Taro Yamane formula, the sample size was calculated to be 474 community pharmacists (333 from Lagos and 141 from Oyo States) [32]. A multistage sampling method was utilized, stratifying pharmacies into zonal arrangements and randomly selecting zones and pharmacies within those zones. Registered pharmacists from the selected pharmacies were surveyed [31].

4. *Data collection methods:* A semi-structured, self-administered questionnaire was used, adapted from previous studies, and validated for the Nigerian context [33–35]. The questionnaire included demographic questions and a 5-point Likert scale to assess perceptions, benefits, and barriers. Data were collected through both paper forms and Google Forms, with follow-ups to maximize response rates. Statistical analysis was performed using SPSS (version 23), with descriptive and inferential statistics (Chi-square, t-tests, and ANOVA) applied [36].

2.1.2 Description of vaccination services and policy advocacy

The study also focused on how community pharmacies delivered vaccination services during the COVID-19 pandemic, evaluating improvements in vaccination coverage. The findings aim to support advocacy for policy changes to officially recognize community pharmacists in immunization service delivery in Nigeria.

2.1.2.1 Qualitative methodology

1. *Study design:* Exploratory in-depth interviews were conducted to gather detailed insights from key stakeholders about community pharmacy vaccination services.

2. *Sampling strategy:* Purposive sampling was used to select key stakeholders, including leaders from the National Primary Health Care Development Agency (NPHCDA), the Association of Community Pharmacists of Nigeria (ACPN), the Pharmacy Council of Nigeria (PCN), and representatives from international organizations like Medicines, Technologies, and Pharmaceutical Services (MTaPS). Consent was obtained from all interviewees.

3. *Data collection methods:* Semi-structured interviews were carried out, some face-to-face and others via email, depending on participants' availability. The interviews were recorded, transcribed, and analyzed using thematic analysis to identify recurring themes and insights. Multiple researchers reviewed the transcripts to ensure reliability and consistency.

2.1.3 Ethical considerations

Ethical approval was obtained from the Oyo State Research Ethical Review Committee, Ministry of Health (Reference No. NHREC/OYOSHRIEC/10/11/22).

Written informed consent was secured from all participants, ensuring voluntary participation and confidentiality. Data were anonymized and securely stored, with access limited to authorized research personnel only.

2.2 Delivery of vaccination services in community pharmacies

2.2.1 Description of vaccination services in Nigerian community pharmacies

In Nigeria, community pharmacies have typically focused on dispensing medications and delivery of basic healthcare services. However, with their expanded role in health promotion, they have included vaccination services, though with few restrictions. Community pharmacies provide various vaccination services including:

1. *Client education:* Pharmacists educate their clients about the benefits and potential side effects of vaccines, making a difference in addressing vaccine hesitancy and misinformation [17, 37].

2. *Vaccine administration:* Community pharmacies are now given the authority to administer COVID-19 vaccines, while others give vaccines covering all ranges of diseases like tetanus, rabies, measles, polio, and Hepatitis-B and others on request [37, 38].

3. *Documentation:* Record keeping of administered vaccines is being maintained for future reference and follow-up, although this practice can be inconsistent.

4. *Referral services:* Referral to other health facilities are made for clients with specific needs or vaccines requiring special storage [17, 37].

Despite these endeavors, the full potential of community pharmacies in vaccination delivery is often compelled by insufficient training, infrastructure limitations, and insufficient policy support [30, 38, 39].

2.2.2 Case study: COVID-19 vaccination experience

The COVID-19 pandemic marked a significant shift in the role of community pharmacies in Nigeria's vaccination efforts. Key aspects include:

1. *Rapid response:* Community pharmacies played a crucial role in the rapid distribution of COVID-19 vaccines. They utilized their accessibility and established patient relationships to facilitate vaccination campaigns [39].

2. *Vaccination administration:* Pharmacies managed vaccine distribution and administration, adhering to stringent cold chain requirements for COVID-19 vaccines [10].

3. *Collaboration:* Through the community pharmacy association, increased collaboration with national and state government PHC agencies allowed pharmacies to integrate into national vaccination strategies, including public health campaigns and vaccination drives [10, 39, 40].

2.2.3 Successes, challenges, and lessons learned

2.2.3.1 Successes

1. *Increased accessibility:* Community pharmacies enhanced vaccine accessibility, particularly in underserved areas with limited healthcare infrastructure. This was significant for improving vaccine coverage [10, 37].

2. *Efficiency and speed:* The flexibility of pharmacies enabled swift vaccine deployment and distribution, leveraging their existing structure and patient networks [10].

3. *Enhanced public trust:* The involvement of community pharmacists helped build public trust in vaccines, as pharmacists were seen as trusted healthcare providers [10, 39].

2.2.3.2 Challenges

1. *Infrastructure limitations:* Many pharmacies struggled with inadequate facilities for vaccine storage and handling, especially with the cold chain prerequisites for COVID-19 vaccines [23].

2. *Training and resources:* The inadequate training and resources for managing COVID-19 vaccines highlighted gaps in preparedness and training among community pharmacists [41].

3. *Policy and regulation:* Vague or insufficient policies for community pharmacy participation in vaccination led to irregularities in vaccine administration and documentation [30, 39].

2.2.3.3 Lessons learned

1. *Need for training:* An all-inclusive training for pharmacists on vaccine administration and emergency response is critical to enhance effectiveness in future vaccination efforts [41].

2. *Infrastructure investment:* Investment in pharmacy infrastructure, particularly for vaccine storage and handling, is necessary for managing future vaccination campaigns [42, 43].

3. *Policy development:* Development of clear and supportive policies to integrate community pharmacies into national vaccination strategies and routine immunization is crucial. This should include guidelines for administration, reimbursement, and quality assurance [30, 39].

The COVID-19 vaccination experience demonstrated the critical role of community pharmacies in public health initiatives. By addressing identified challenges and building on successes, community pharmacies can become a more integral part of Nigeria's healthcare system, particularly in enhancing vaccination coverage and responding to future public health emergencies [5].

3. Findings and analysis

3.1 Summary of quantitative results

Demographics and response rate: A total of 411 community pharmacists from Lagos and Oyo States, Nigeria, participated in the study, with a response rate of 86.7%. Most respondents were from Lagos (72.0%) and had a mean age of 43.06 years. The majority were male, and held a B.Pharm/B.Sc. Pharm degree, and worked in independent pharmacies. Pharmacy owners constituted 52.6% of the respondents, with 42.6% having 1–10 years of postgraduation experience.

Vaccination training and services provided: Less than half of the respondents (40.1%) had undergone vaccination training, primarily through pharmacy professional associations, NGOs, and webinars. A smaller proportion (31.4%) provided vaccination services, with activities including patient education, referrals, vaccine administration, and storage.

Statistical analysis and correlations: There were significant differences between respondents from Lagos and Oyo States in mean age, postgraduation experience, and community pharmacy experience. Significant associations were also found regarding the type of pharmacy and employment status, but not with gender, degree, vaccination training, or services provided.

Perceptions of vaccination services: Over 90% of respondents supported the role of community pharmacies in administering vaccines, inclusion in the national database, and granting authority to administer vaccines. A statistically significant difference was observed in the perception that community pharmacists should be given the authority to administer vaccines between the two states.

Perceived benefits of community pharmacies as vaccination centers: Respondents overwhelmingly agreed that using community pharmacies as vaccination centers would improve vaccination coverage, increase accessibility, and enhance pharmaceutical care. There was a significant difference in the perception of improving vaccination coverage in Nigeria between the two states.

Potential barriers to providing vaccination services: Less than half of the respondents identified barriers such as increased workload, lack of client demand, and lack of private areas. However, more than 50% agreed that lack of government authorization, collaboration, and inadequate training were significant barriers.

Correlations and differences: There was a strong positive correlation between overall perceived benefits and perceptions of vaccination services in community pharmacies. In contrast, the correlation between perceived benefits and potential barriers was weak and positive, and the correlation between barriers and perceptions was weak and negative.

Factors associated with perception, benefits, and barriers: Significant factors influencing perceptions included the state of practice, employment status, vaccination training, level of education, and provision of vaccination services. Similar factors were associated with perceived benefits and potential barriers.

Service provision details: Of the 72 respondents who administered vaccines, 62.5% had experience with vaccine administration prior to COVID-19. The majority of the vaccinators were pharmacists (79.2%), followed by registered trained nurses (29.2%) and community health workers (13.9%). Most (83.3%) administered vaccines upon request, 30.6% only administered COVID-19 vaccines, and only 9.7% had administered over 500 doses of the COVID-19 vaccine (**Table 1**).

Response theme (N = 72)	Total freq. (%)
I administered vaccines before COVID-19 pandemic in my pharmacy	45 (70.6)
Health personnel who administer the vaccines in my pharmacy	
Registered trained nurse	21 (29.2)
Auxiliary nurse	9 (12.5)
CHEW	10 (13.9)
Pharmacy technician	3 (4.2)
Pharmacists	57 (79.1)
Other healthcare professionals in the pharmacy	7 (9.7)
Types of vaccines administered:	
Routine immunization for children	6 (8.3)
COVID-19 vaccine	22 (30.6)
All range of vaccines	14 (19.4)
Vaccines on request	60 (83.3)
Number of COVID-19 vaccine doses administered	
1–100	6 (8.3)
101–500	5 (6.9)
501–1000	3 (4.2)
>1000	4 (5.6)

Table 1.
Response from those administering vaccines in their pharmacies ONLY (N = 72).

Logistic regression analysis: A logistic regression analysis was conducted to assess factors influencing the provision of vaccination services by community pharmacists (**Table 2**). The training was statistically significant (p = 0.000), showing that pharmacists who had received vaccination training were approximately eight times more likely to provide vaccination services compared to those who had not been trained (coefficient = 2.120, 95% CI: 5.043–13.770). Other variables, including employment status (p = 0.270), highest level of education (p = 0.092), years of postgraduation experience (p = 0.054), years of community pharmacy practice (p = 0.645), and age (p = 0.225), did not show significant effects.

Suggestions for improvement: Respondents suggested enhancing vaccination coverage through government support, inclusion of pharmacists in the national database, recognition as primary healthcare providers, further training, and provision of adequate facilities for vaccination projects.

3.2 Qualitative results

The thematic analysis of the in-depth interviews with key stakeholders produced five main themes, each shedding light on different aspects of vaccination services provided by community pharmacists (CPs) and the associated challenges and opportunities.

Variable	Coefficient	p-Value	Exp (B)	95% CI	
N = 411				**Lower**	**Upper**
Employment status					
Employee pharmacists		Reference category			
Pharmacist owners	0.325	0.270	1.384	0.777	2.464
Undergone vaccination training					
No		Reference category			
Yes	2.120	0.000*	8.334	5.043	13.770
Level of education					
Ph.D.		Reference category 0.092			
B. Pharm	0.908	0.465ns	2.478	0.217	28.351
Pharm. D	0.034	0.980ns	1.035	0.070	15.218
Master's degrees/PGDs	0.427	0.734ns	1.533	0.130	18.042
Fellow WAPCP	1.649	0.208ns	5.200	0.400	67.677
Age (in years)	0.040	0.225ns	1.041	0.976	1.111
Year of experience postgraduation	−0.069	0.054ns	0.933	0.869	1.001
Year of experience in community pharmacy practice	0.011	0.645ns	1.011	0.964	1.060
Constant	−0.3467	0.021	0.031		

*Significant at ≤0.05 p-value.
ns is not significant. CI: confidence interval.

Table 2.
Predictors of vaccination services provided by community pharmacists.

3.2.1 Theme 1: Perspectives on the effect of vaccination skills training among community pharmacists

Stakeholders uniformly viewed vaccination skills training as highly beneficial. A major stakeholder from a pharmacy professional association described the training as:

> *"The opportunity for CPs to improve their knowledge; improve skills of members as registered vaccinators; improve access to vaccines to the public as CPs are easily accessible and trusted by their clients."*

The training's positive impact on public health was highlighted, with improved competence among CPs leading to enhanced management of diseases such as TB and HIV/AIDS. Stakeholders noted:

> *"Clients are happy and highly excited that CPs can vaccinate them. It is convenient for them."*

A Pharmacy Regulatory Agency leader emphasized the broader public health benefits:

> *"Engagement of community pharmacies will expand access and reduce disease."*

Training CPs was seen as a cost-effective strategy for improving vaccination coverage and public health outcomes:

> *"It will promote access; improve coverage; reduce the cost of individual travel to PHC centers; increase efficiency; reduce the burden of disease... Therefore, it is a welcome development that is hoped to maintain progress in the future."*

3.2.2 Theme 2: Sustainability of vaccination training among pharmacists

The progress of vaccination training programs for CPs was noted with various achievements:

> *"We had trained over 700 CPs in all with NGO's involvement... Over 15,000 vaccines had been administered, and data were captured by MTaPS between August 2022 and January 2023. Oyo State had the largest volume of about 11,000 vaccine doses administered."*

In Lagos State, more than 100 CPs were trained, with over 2000 doses administered through three CPs. In Oyo State, 20 CPs were actively involved in vaccination.

Plans for expansion included integrating vaccination training into the Mandatory Continuing Professional Development modules and leveraging partnerships with international agencies for training and equipment support.

3.2.3 Theme 3: Policy

Current policies were noted to lack formal support for CPs as vaccination centers:

> *"There is no policy against pharmacies serving as vaccination centers, nor is there a policy for pharmacies to serve either... The policy presently does not allow for it."*

However, the engagement of CPs during the COVID-19 pandemic was seen as an innovative solution to increase access. Stakeholders indicated a need for clearer policies and formal agreements:

> *"No law gives CPs the right, but there is an understanding that needs to be formalized between the NPHCDA and the CPs."*

Recommendations included:

> *"Vaccines should be provided free to encourage client vaccination; registered CP vaccinators should be remunerated."*

Efforts to formalize the role of CPs in vaccination services were ongoing, with suggestions for clearer policy frameworks and partnerships.

3.2.4 Theme 4: Community pharmacists' involvement in vaccination

To increase CP involvement, stakeholders proposed strategies such as:

> *"Establishment of Vaccine Advisory Monitoring & Evaluation Committee (VAMEC) to monitor vaccine administration in the CPs" and "Collaborative interventions, such as advocacy with policymakers and government functionaries, e.g., NPHCDA and State PHC boards."*

The potential for CPs to contribute significantly to public health interventions was acknowledged, with calls for recognition and expanded roles:

> *"CPs are ready to provide fee-for-service vaccination as part of their service to the community; CPs are partners in healthcare delivery; they are well-trained but underutilized."*

3.2.5 Theme 5: Challenges

Several challenges were identified, including financial constraints, logistical issues, and limited facilities. Notable challenges included:

> *"Expansion had been limited by inspection processes, the linkage between CPs and PHC Board in 20 Local Government Areas (LGAs) in Lagos State and process of accreditation of facilities by the State PHC Board..."*

Other challenges were related to the cost of vaccine administration and the need for cold chain facilities:

> *"Expansion is limited to funding by the NGO; need for cold chain facilities, as the CPs still pick and return vaccines from PHC centers daily; logistics issues; space in some pharmacies; staffing issues as the process is very demanding."*

The lack of uniform affordability for training among CPs was also a barrier:

> *"Not every CP can pay for the training."*

3.3 Key insights

3.3.1 Vaccination training and service provision

- *Prevalence of training*: Less than half (40.1%) of respondents had undergone vaccination training. The majority of these trainings were provided by professional associations (64.8%) and NGOs (26.1%).

- *Service provision*: Only 31.4% of respondents provided vaccination services. Among these, the most common services included education on vaccination (78.3%), referrals (58.1%), vaccine administration (55.8%), and storage (36.4%).

3.3.2 Characteristics of vaccinators

- *Demographics*: Of the 72 respondents who administered vaccines, a significant proportion (79.2%) were pharmacists, followed by registered nurses (29.2%) and community health workers (13.9%).

- *Vaccination practices*: A majority (83.3%) administered vaccines on request, while only a small fraction had administered over 500 doses of COVID-19 vaccines (9.7%).

3.3.3 Impact of training on service provision

- *Statistical significance*: Training in vaccination services was found to be statistically significant ($p = 0.000$) in relation to the provision of vaccination services. The odds of providing vaccination services were about eight times higher for those who had undergone training.

- *Training effectiveness*: The coefficient of 2.120 (95% CI: 5.043–13.770) indicates a strong positive association between training and the likelihood of providing vaccination services.

3.3.4 Stakeholder perspectives

- *Positive outcomes*: Stakeholders noted that vaccination training improved CPs' knowledge and skills, making them more accessible and trusted by the public. This improved access contributed to better public health outcomes and cost-effectiveness.

- *Sustainability*: Training programs have successfully reached over 700 CPs, with significant vaccine doses administered, particularly in Oyo and Lagos States. Plans are in place to expand training through Mandatory Continuing Professional Development modules and partnerships.

3.3.5 Policy and regulatory issues

- *Current policies*: There is no formal policy supporting or restricting CPs from serving as vaccination centers. The COVID-19 pandemic prompted innovative solutions, but a clear policy framework is still lacking.

- *Recommendations*: Stakeholders recommend formalizing policies to support CP involvement in vaccination, including providing free vaccines, recognizing CPs as primary healthcare providers, and ensuring adequate remuneration for their services.

3.3.6 Challenges and barriers

- *Financial and logistical challenges*: Limited funding, logistical issues, and the need for cold chain facilities were significant barriers. Some CPs faced difficulties in affording training and maintaining facilities.

- *Policy uncertainty*: The lack of a clear policy framework hinders the consistent and widespread involvement of CPs in vaccination services.

3.4 Trends and patterns

3.4.1 Increased training and involvement

- There is a growing trend toward training CPs in vaccination services, with increasing numbers of CPs becoming actively involved in vaccine administration. This reflects a shift toward utilizing community pharmacies as vaccination sites.

3.4.2 Policy and regulation evolution

- The evolving role of CPs in vaccination, particularly during emergencies like the COVID-19 pandemic, highlights a trend toward exploring and potentially formalizing their involvement through policy changes.

3.4.3 Ongoing challenges

- Persistent challenges related to funding, logistical support, and policy clarity continue to affect the effectiveness and sustainability of vaccination services provided by CPs.

4. Impact and implications

1. *Improvement in vaccination coverage:* The research findings underscore the significant impact of vaccination training on community pharmacists' (CPs) ability to provide vaccination services. The statistically significant association between training and service provision demonstrates the crucial role of equipping CPs with the necessary skills and knowledge. This association indicates that CPs who receive vaccination training are approximately eight times more likely to offer vaccination services compared to those who do not.

   Increased service availability: Training enables CPs to administer vaccines, educate patients, and manage vaccination logistics effectively. This expanded role enhances access to vaccination services, particularly in underserved areas where CPs are more accessible than traditional healthcare facilities [8, 39]. The provision of vaccines by CPs helps bridge gaps in vaccination coverage, leading to higher overall immunization rates in the community [10, 41, 44].
   Enhanced vaccine delivery: The involvement of CPs in vaccine administration improves convenience for patients, leading to increased vaccination uptake. The positive feedback from the community regarding the ease of accessing vaccinations through CPs indicates a higher likelihood of timely vaccination [8]. This increased accessibility supports higher vaccination rates, especially in regions with limited healthcare infrastructure [6].
   Recognition of the pharmacy association's efforts: The inclusion of community pharmacists in COVID-19 vaccination efforts in Nigeria was significantly bolstered by the strategic training initiatives spearheaded by the Community Pharmacy Association. These training programs played a pivotal role in equipping pharmacists with the necessary skills and knowledge, enabling them to actively participate in the national vaccination campaign. This initiative not only expanded the reach of vaccination services but also highlighted the critical role of pharmacists in public health, particularly during a global health crisis [40, 45].

2. *Community acceptance and public health outcomes:* The integration of CPs into vaccination efforts has favorable implications for community acceptance and

public health outcomes. Stakeholders have noted that the presence of CPs as vaccinators is well-received, which enhances the overall acceptance of vaccination programs [39].

Public perception and trust: The positive reception of CPs by the community reflects their role as trusted healthcare providers. Many respondents expressed satisfaction with the convenience of receiving vaccinations from CPs, which correlates with higher adherence rates and positive health outcomes [46]. The reduced barriers to immunization facilitated by CPs contribute to improved public health [5].
Health outcomes: The involvement of CPs in vaccination services leads to improved health outcomes by increasing vaccine coverage and preventing diseases. Stakeholders have highlighted that broader vaccination coverage through CPs results in reduced disease incidence and enhanced public health [1, 39]. This expanded access not only prevents individual illness but also contributes to community-wide immunity, ultimately reducing the burden of infectious diseases [30].

3. *Policy implications and recommendations:* The research highlights several policy implications and recommendations for optimizing the role of CPs in vaccination services.

Need for policy development: The current lack of formal policies supporting or regulating CPs as vaccination providers creates uncertainty and limits their potential impact. There is a clear need for comprehensive policies that formalize and support the role of CPs in vaccination services. Such policies should address issues related to training, remuneration, and facility accreditation [8, 30, 39].

Recommendations for policy changes:

- *Formal recognition and support:* Policies should officially recognize CPs as key providers of vaccination services. This recognition can lead to structured integration into national vaccination programs and ensure inclusion in the national health database [44].

- *Financial and logistical support:* Government and regulatory bodies should provide financial support for CPs to facilitate training and facility upgrades. This includes funding for cold chain facilities and logistics to ensure effective vaccine administration [5].

- *Regulatory framework:* Establishing a clear regulatory framework outlining responsibilities and standards for CPs involved in vaccination is essential. This framework should include guidelines for training, vaccine storage, and administration practices [47].

Future directions:

- *Collaboration with stakeholders:* Ongoing collaboration between government agencies, professional associations, and NGOs is crucial for successful policy implementation and program support. Partnerships can aid in training programs, equipment provision, and resource allocation for CPs.

- *Evaluation and adaptation:* Continuous evaluation of CPs' impact on vaccination coverage and public health outcomes is necessary. Policymakers should adopt strategies based on feedback and emerging data to optimize CP involvement in vaccination efforts.

By addressing these policy implications and recommendations, stakeholders can enhance the role of CPs in vaccination services, improve vaccination coverage, and ultimately achieve better public health outcomes.

5. Conclusion

5.1 Recap of key points

This study provides a comprehensive examination of the current landscape of vaccination services delivered by community pharmacists in Nigeria. The findings reveal several critical insights:

- *Training and service delivery*: Less than half of the respondents had undergone vaccination training, with the most common sources being professional associations and NGOs. Despite this, a significant proportion of community pharmacists are involved in providing vaccination services, including education, referrals, vaccine administration, and storage.

- *Impact of training*: Logistic regression analysis demonstrated that vaccination training significantly enhances the likelihood of community pharmacists providing vaccination services, with trained pharmacists being approximately eight times more likely to offer these services compared to their untrained counterparts.

- *Qualitative insights*: Stakeholder interviews highlighted the positive impact of training on public health outcomes, emphasizing increased accessibility and cost-effectiveness. However, challenges such as policy gaps, financial constraints, and logistical issues remain.

- *Policy and practice*: Current policies are not fully supportive of community pharmacies as vaccination centers, though recent emergency situations have showcased their potential. Recommendations include formalizing policy support and enhancing training and resources for pharmacists.

5.2 Future directions and potential for further research

Future research should address the following areas:

1. *Policy development*: Investigating how policy can better support the integration of community pharmacists into vaccination services and exploring models from other countries could provide valuable insights.

2. *Training programs*: Assessing the long-term impact of vaccination training programs on service delivery and public health outcomes will be crucial for refining and scaling these initiatives.

3. *Public perception*: Understanding community attitudes toward pharmacists as vaccinators and identifying barriers to acceptance can help tailor strategies to improve vaccine uptake.

4. *Resource allocation*: Researching effective ways to address logistical and financial challenges, including cold chain management and funding mechanisms, will be important for expanding the role of community pharmacists in vaccination services.

By addressing these areas, future research can contribute to a more robust and effective vaccination strategy in Nigeria, leveraging community pharmacists' unique position to enhance public health.

6. Summary

This chapter has explored the critical role of community pharmacists (CPs) in enhancing vaccination coverage, particularly in the context of Nigeria's healthcare landscape. The findings underscore the significant impact of targeted training programs on CPs' ability to provide vaccination services, leading to increased service availability and improved public health outcomes.

The evidence presented demonstrates that well-trained CPs are crucial in bridging the gap in vaccination coverage, especially in underserved areas where traditional healthcare facilities are less accessible. By involving CPs in vaccination efforts, communities benefit from greater convenience, higher vaccine uptake, and ultimately, better protection against vaccine-preventable diseases.

Furthermore, the positive reception of CPs as vaccinators highlights their trusted position within the community, which fosters higher acceptance of vaccination programs. This trust, coupled with the strategic inclusion of CPs in public health initiatives, has the potential to significantly enhance overall immunization rates and reduce the burden of infectious diseases.

The chapter also outlines essential policy recommendations to optimize the role of CPs in vaccination services. These include the need for formal recognition and support of CPs as key providers of vaccination, financial and logistical backing, and the establishment of a clear regulatory framework. Collaboration among stakeholders, continuous evaluation, and adaptation of strategies are critical to sustaining and improving the impact of CPs on vaccination efforts.

In recognizing the efforts of professional bodies like the Pharmacy Association in training their members, this chapter acknowledges that such initiatives are vital for the successful integration of CPs into national vaccination strategies. The inclusion of CPs in COVID-19 vaccination efforts in Nigeria serves as a testament to the effectiveness of these training programs and sets a precedent for future public health interventions.

In conclusion, by leveraging the capabilities of community pharmacists through comprehensive training and supportive policies, Nigeria can achieve higher vaccination coverage, better public health outcomes, and a stronger, more resilient healthcare system.

Acknowledgements

The author acknowledges the use of ChatGPT for the language polishing of the manuscript.

Author details

Yejide Olukemi Oseni
Department of Clinical Pharmacy and Pharmacy Administration, Faculty of Pharmacy, Lead City University, Ibadan, Nigeria

*Address all correspondence to: yejideoseni@yahoo.com; oseni.yejide@lcu.edu.ng

References

[1] World Health Organisation (WHO). Immunization Coverage. 2024. Available from: https://www.who.int/news-room/factsheets/detail/immunization-coverage

[2] Mistry SK, Ali AM, Yadav UN, Huda MN, Parray AA, Mahumud RA, et al. COVID-19 vaccination coverage is extremely low among older population in Bangladesh: Findings from a cross-sectional study. Human Vaccines & Immunotherapeutics. 2022;**18**(1):2030624. DOI: 10.1080/21645515.2022.2030624. Epub 2022 Feb 17

[3] Moyazzem Hossain M, Abdulla F, Rahman A. Challenges and difficulties faced in low- and middle-income countries during COVID-19. Health Policy OPEN. 2022;**3**(2022):100082. Epub 2022 Nov 8. DOI: 10.1016/j.hpopen.2022.100082

[4] Adigwe OP, Oturu D, Onavbavba G. Healthcare professionals' views on access to vaccines in Nigeria: A cross sectional study. Vaccine X. 2022;**12**:100235. DOI: 10.1016/j.jvacx.2022.100235

[5] Berenbrok LA, Tang S, Gabriel N, et al. Access to community pharmacies: A nationwide geographic information systems cross-sectional analysis. Journal of the American Pharmaceutical Association. 2022;**62**(6):1816-1822.e2. DOI: 10.1016/j.japh.2022.07.003

[6] Stämpfli D, Martinez-De la Torre A, Simi E, Du Pasquier S, Berger J, Burden AM. Community pharmacist-administered COVID-19 vaccinations: A pilot customer survey on satisfaction and motivation to get vaccinated. Vaccines (Basel). 2021;**9**(11):1320. DOI: 10.3390/vaccines9111320

[7] Percy JN, Crain J, Rein L, Hohmeier KC. The impact of a pharmacist-extender training program to improve pneumococcal vaccination rates within a community chain pharmacy. Journal of the American Pharmaceutical Association. 2020;**60**(1):39-46

[8] Le LM, Veettil SK, Donaldson D, et al. The impact of pharmacist involvement on immunization uptake and other outcomes: An updated systematic review and meta-analysis. Journal of the American Pharmaceutical Association. 2022;**62**(5):1499-1513.e16. DOI: 10.1016/j.japh.2022.06.008

[9] Alnahar SA, Gkountouras G, Darwish RM, Bates I. Community pharmacists workforce readiness to deliver vaccination services: A cross-sectional study from Jordan. Pharmacology Research & Perspectives. 2022;**10**(2). DOI: 10.1002/prp2.943

[10] Edoziem V, Umar-Farouk O, Omolara O. Improving Demand Generation for Covid-19 Vaccination through Privately Owned Community Pharmacies. Breakthrough ACTION and Breakthrough RESEARCH/USAID; 2023. Available from: https://breakthroughactionandresearch.org/improving-covid-19-vaccine-demand-through-pharmacies/

[11] Christian BN, Christian NG, Keshinro MI, Olutade-Babatunde O. How to build bridges for universal health coverage in Nigeria by linking formal and informal health providers. BMJ Global Health. 2023;**8**(11):e014165. DOI: 10.1136/bmjgh-2023-014165

[12] Federal Ministry of Health. National Health Policy. 2020. Available from: https://www.moh.gov.gh/wp-content/uploads/2021/08/NHP_January-2020.pdf

[13] Gyuse AN, Ayuk AE, Okeke MC. Facilitators and barriers to effective primary health care in Nigeria. African Journal of Primary Health Care & Family Medicine. 2018;**10**(1):e1-e3. DOI: 10.4102/phcfm.v10i1.1641

[14] Amaeze OU, Akinola AA, Aiyeolemi AA, Lawal FO, Ijomone OR, Mbata UA. Community Pharmacists' Services during the COVID-19 pandemic: A case study of Lagos State, Nigeria. Journal of Research in Pharmacy Practice. 2022;**11**(1):25-32. DOI: 10.4103/jrpp.jrpp_5_22Adigw

[15] Nwankwo ONO, Ugwu CI, Nwankwo GI, Akpoke MA, Anyigor C, Obi-Nwankwo U, et al. A qualitative inquiry of rural-urban inequalities in the distribution and retention of healthcare workers in southern Nigeria. PLoS ONE. 2022;**17**(3):e0266159. DOI: 10.1371/journal.pone.0266159

[16] Babatope T, Ilyenkova V, Marais D. COVID-19 vaccine hesitancy: A systematic review of barriers to the uptake of COVID-19 vaccine among adults in Nigeria. Bulletin of the National Research Centre. 2023;**47**(1):45. DOI: 10.1186/s42269-023-01017-w. Epub 2023 Mar 21

[17] Adesola RO, Opuni E, Idris I, Okesanya OJ, Igwe O, Abdulazeez MD, et al. Navigating Nigeria's health landscape: Population growth and its health implications. Environmental Health Insights. 2024;**18**:11786302241250211. DOI: 10.1177/11786302241250211

[18] Aderemi-Williams RI, Igwilo CI. Community pharmacies as possible centres for routine immunization. Nigerian Quarterly Journal of Hospital Medicine. 2007;**17**(4):131-133. DOI: 10.4314/nqjhm.v17i4.12692

[19] NPHCDA. Goals of NPHCDA National Primary Health Care Development Agency. 2024. Available from: https://nphcda.gov.ng/services/

[20] WHO. Vaccines and Immunization. World Health Organisation; 2024. Available from: https://www.who.int/health-topics/vaccines-and-immunization#tab=tab_1

[21] WHO. Polio Eradication Initiative: Immunization. 2024. Available from: https://www.emro.who.int/polio-eradication/about-eradication/immunization.html#:~:text=Mass%20immunization%20campaigns%2C%20known%20as,a%20child%20follows%20from%20birth

[22] Voorman A, Lyons H, Shuaib F, Adamu US, Korir C, Erbeto T, et al. Impact of supplementary immunization activities using novel oral polio vaccine type 2 during a large outbreak of circulating vaccine-derived poliovirus in Nigeria. The Journal of Infectious Diseases. 2024;**229**(3):805-812. DOI: 10.1093/infdis/jiad222

[23] Olutuase VO, Iwu-Jaja CJ, Akuoko CP, Adewuyi EO, Khanal V. Medicines and vaccines supply chains challenges in Nigeria: A scoping review. BMC Public Health. 2022;**22**(1):11. DOI: 10.1186/s12889-021-12361-9

[24] Gibson E, Zameer M, Alban R, Kouwanou LM. Community health workers as vaccinators: A rapid review of the global landscape, 2000-2021. Global Health: Science and Practice. 2023;**11**(1):e2200307. DOI: 10.9745/GHSP-D-22-00307

[25] Galagali PM, Kinikar AA, Kumar VS. Vaccine hesitancy: Obstacles and challenges. Current Pediatrics Reports. 2022;**10**(4):241-248. DOI: 10.1007/s40124-022-00278-9 Epub 2022 Oct 8

[26] Ekezie W, Awwad S, Krauchenberg A, Karara N, Dembiński Ł, Grossman Z, et al. Access to vaccination among disadvantaged, isolated and difficult-to-reach communities in the WHO European Region: A systematic review. Vaccines (Basel). 2022;**10**(7):1038. DOI: 10.3390/vaccines10071038

[27] Goode JV, Owen J, Page A, Gatewood S. Community-based pharmacy practice innovation and the role of the community-based pharmacist practitioner in the United States. Pharmacy (Basel). 2019;**7**(3):106. DOI: 10.3390/pharmacy7030106

[28] Bach AT, Goad JA. The role of community pharmacy-based vaccination in the USA: Current practice and future directions. Integrated Pharmacy Research and Practice. 2015;**4**:67-77. DOI: 10.2147/IPRP.S63822

[29] Romero-Mancilla MS, Mora-Vargas J, Ruiz A. Pharmacy-based immunization: A systematic review. Frontiers in Public Health. 2023;**11**:1152556. DOI: 10.3389/fpubh.2023.1152556

[30] Wada YH, Musa MK, Ekpenyong A, Adebisi YA, Musa MB, Khalid GM. Increasing coverage of vaccination by pharmacists in Nigeria; an urgent need. Public Health in Practice. 2021;**2**:100148

[31] Pharmacy Council of Nigeria (PCN) Register of Pharmacists and Pharmaceutical Premises as at December 31, 2022. 2022

[32] Yamane T. Statistics: An Introductory Analysis. 2nd ed. New York: Harper and Row; 1967

[33] Tadele S, Demissie BN, Tamiru MT, Tadesse TA. Knowledge and attitudes of community pharmacists on vaccination, barriers and willingness to implement community pharmacy-based vaccination services in Ethiopia. Human Vaccines & Immunotherapeutics. 2023;**19**(3):2291243. DOI: 10.1080/21645515.2023.2291243

[34] Jarab AS, Al-Qerem W, Mukattash TL. Community pharmacists' willingness and barriers to provide vaccination during COVID-19 pandemic in Jordan. Human Vaccines & Immunotherapeutics. 2022;**18**(1):2016009. DOI: 10.1080/21645515.2021.2016009

[35] Turcu-Stiolica A, Kamusheva M, Bogdan M, Tadic I, Harasani K, Subtirelu MS, et al. Pharmacist's perspectives on administering a COVID-19 vaccine in community pharmacies in four Balkan countries. Frontiers in Public Health. 2021;**9**:766146. DOI: 10.3389/fpubh.2021.766146

[36] SPSS Inc. SPSS Statistics Version 23. SPSS Inc.; 2023

[37] Oseni YO, Okafor UG, et al. Improving vaccination coverage through community pharmacy service delivery in Nigeria; the COVID-19 experience and implications for policy review. Health Care Science. 2024. (under review)

[38] Agbo BB, Esienumoh E, Inah SA, Eko JE, Nwachukwu EJ. Community pharmacists' participation in immunization services in Cross River State, Nigeria. International Journal of Public Health, Pharmacy and Pharmacology. 2019;**4**(3):11-25. Available from: https://eajournals.org/ijphpp/vol-4-issue-3-august-2019/community-pharmacists-participation-in-immunization-services-in-cross-river-state-nigeria/

[39] Okafor UG, Oseni YO, Odukoya TO, et al. Stakeholders' perspectives on involvement of community pharmacists

in vaccine delivery services and implications for policy reform in Nigeria. Discover Public Health. 2024;**21**:26. DOI: 10.1186/s12982-024-00151-8

[40] Adebowale-Tambe N. COVID-19: Nigerian govt partners community pharmacies to expand vaccination coverage, May 31, 2022. The Premium Times. 2022

[41] Enejoh D. Strategizing for Results: Mobilizing the Private Sector for COVID-19 Response in Nigeria. Medicines, Technologies, and Pharmaceutical Services (MTaPS); 2023. Available from: https://www.mtapsprogram.org/news-blog/strategizing-for-results-mobilizing-the-private-sector-for-covid-19-response-in-nigeria/#:~:text=By%20the%20end%20of%20the,COVID%2D19%20program%20in%20Nigeria

[42] Ayenew W, Anagaw YK, Limenh LW, Simegn W, Bizuneh GK, Bitew T, et al. Readiness of and barriers for community pharmacy professionals in providing and implementing vaccination services. BMC Health Services Research. 2024;**24**(1):867. DOI: 10.1186/s12913-024-11349-6

[43] Padula WV, Malaviya S, Reid NM, Cohen BG, Chingcuanco F, Ballreich J, et al. Economic value of vaccines to address the COVID-19 pandemic: A U.S. cost-effectiveness and budget impact analysis. Journal of Medical Economics. 2021;**24**(1):1060-1069. DOI: 10.1080/13696998.2021.1965732

[44] Yemeke TT, McMillan S, Marciniak MW, Ozawa S. A systematic review of the role of pharmacists in vaccination services in low-and middle-income countries. Research in Social & Administrative Pharmacy. 2021;**17**(2):300-306. DOI: 10.1016/j.sapharm.2020.03.016

[45] Ojerinde D. PSN, ACPN hail inclusion of community pharmacies as vaccination centres, November 17, 2021. The PUNCH Newspaper. 2021

[46] Merks P, Kowalczuk A, Wong A, Chung K, Religioni U, Świetlik D, et al. Patient satisfaction with pharmacist-administered COVID-19 vaccines in Poland: A survey study in the vaccination centres context. BMC Health Services Research. 2022;**22**(1):1339. DOI: 10.1186/s12913-022-08720-w

[47] International Pharmaceutical Federation (FIP). FIP Commitments to Action: FIP Commitment to Accelerating Vaccination Equity, Access and Sustainability through Pharmacy. 2021. Available from: https://transformingvaccination.fip.org/2021-fip-commitment-to-action/

Chapter 5

The Role of Preventive Health Care in Preventing Chronic Diseases

Gudeta D. Fufaa

Abstract

Preventive health care is essential in reducing the prevalence and impact of chronic diseases, which are major causes of death and illness worldwide. Chronic diseases like cardiovascular disease, diabetes, cancer, and respiratory conditions result from genetic, lifestyle, and environmental factors. This document explores these risk factors and highlights the importance of preventive strategies at primary, secondary, and tertiary levels. Primary prevention focuses on avoiding disease onset through lifestyle changes and policy measures, while secondary prevention emphasizes early detection and treatment. Tertiary prevention aims to manage and reduce complications in those with chronic conditions. Health care providers play a crucial role through patient education, early detection, and a multidisciplinary approach. Public policies, such as tobacco control and nutrition policies, are vital for fostering healthier communities. However, challenges like socioeconomic disparities and limited access to preventive services hinder effective implementation. Addressing these obstacles through targeted policy interventions, community involvement, and culturally sensitive care is crucial. Future research should focus on the impact of telehealth, health coverage expansions, digital health literacy, social determinants of health, and integrated care models.

Keywords: access to health care, chronic diseases, environmental influences, genetic, predisposition, lifestyle choices, prevention strategies, preventive health care, public policy and chronic diseases

1. Introduction

The application of healthcare measures to prevent diseases is described as preventive health care. Preventive health care plays a crucial role in preventing and managing chronic diseases. Chronic diseases are generally described as conditions that persist for a year or longer and necessitate continuous medical care or restrict daily activities, or both [1]. Chronic diseases, such as heart disease, diabetes, respiratory diseases, and cancer, are among the leading causes of death and disability worldwide [2]. The significance of preventive health care includes a reduction in the incidence of diseases, early detection of risk factors or early stages of chronic diseases, reduction of the long-term costs associated with treating advanced stages of chronic diseases, reduced absenteeism from work and increased productivity, improved physical and mental well-being, reduced risk of health complications, increased life-expectancy, empowerment of individuals and communities, and reduction in health disparities. Prevention of chronic diseases calls for the identification of risk factors at both individual and population levels. The risk factors for chronic diseases can broadly be classified into genetic predisposition, lifestyle choices, and environmental influences.

2. Genetic predisposition

2.1 Cardiovascular disease

Cardiovascular disease (CVD) encompasses a range of conditions affecting the heart and blood vessels, including coronary artery disease, hypertension, and stroke. Numerous studies have identified genetic variants associated with increased CVD risk. A landmark study by Kathiresan et al. [3] utilized genome-wide association studies (GWAS) to identify several loci linked to myocardial infarction. The study found that individuals carrying multiple risk alleles at these loci had a significantly higher risk of heart attacks, independent of traditional risk factors such as diet and lifestyle. Similarly, the Framingham Heart Study [4] highlighted the heritability of CVD, suggesting that genetic factors account for a substantial portion of the variation in CVD risk among individuals.

2.2 Diabetes mellitus

Type 2 diabetes mellitus (T2DM) is another chronic disease with a strong genetic component. Genome-wide association studies have identified numerous genetic variants associated with T2DM risk, many of which are involved in pancreatic beta-cell function and insulin resistance. A study by Voight et al. [5] identified over 30 genetic loci associated with T2DM, emphasizing the polygenic nature of the disease. The Diabetes Prevention Program (DPP) further demonstrated that individuals with a family history of diabetes are at a higher risk of developing T2DM, underscoring the role of genetic predisposition [6].

2.3 Cancer

Genetic predisposition to cancer has been extensively studied, with certain hereditary syndromes, such as Lynch syndrome and BRCA mutations, being well-documented. These genetic mutations significantly increase the risk of specific cancers, including colorectal, breast, and ovarian cancers. According to a study by Miki et al. [7], BRCA1 and BRCA2 mutations confer a markedly increased risk of breast and ovarian cancers. The study highlighted that individuals with these mutations have a lifetime risk of up to 80% for breast cancer and 40% for ovarian cancer. Similarly, Lynch syndrome, caused by mutations in mismatch repair genes, is associated with a high risk of colorectal cancer [8].

2.4 Chronic respiratory diseases

Chronic respiratory diseases, such as asthma, chronic obstructive pulmonary disease (COPD), and cystic fibrosis (CF), pose significant health burdens worldwide.

Asthma is a complex respiratory condition characterized by chronic inflammation and hyperreactivity of the airways. Genetic predisposition to asthma has been extensively studied, with numerous genes identified as contributors to the disease. A study by Ober and Hoffjan [9] reviewed the genetic basis of asthma, identifying over 100 genes associated with the condition. These genes are involved in immune response regulation, airway remodeling, and inflammatory processes. Another notable study by Moffatt et al. [10] identified a locus on chromosome 17q21 that is strongly associated with childhood asthma. This locus includes the ORMDL3 gene, which is implicated in the regulation of inflammation and airway hyperresponsiveness. COPD is a progressive respiratory disease characterized by airflow limitation and chronic inflammation. Genetic factors, in addition to environmental exposures like smoking, contribute to the development and progression of COPD. The most well-known genetic risk factor for COPD is the deficiency of alpha-1 antitrypsin (AAT), a protein that protects the lungs from inflammation-induced damage. Genetic mutations in the SERPINA1 gene lead to AAT deficiency, significantly increasing the risk of developing COPD [11]. Additionally, GWAS have identified several other genetic loci associated with COPD susceptibility, including the CHRNA3/5 locus, which is linked to nicotine addiction and lung function [12]. Cystic fibrosis (CF) is a hereditary disorder caused by mutations in the CFTR gene, which encodes the cystic fibrosis transmembrane conductance regulator protein. This protein is crucial for regulating the movement of chloride and sodium ions across epithelial cells, affecting the mucus consistency in the lungs. Kerem et al. [13] discovered that mutations in the CFTR gene are responsible for CF, with the ΔF508 mutation being the most common. Individuals with CF inherit two defective copies of the CFTR gene, leading to severe respiratory and digestive problems. The identification of CFTR mutations has enabled genetic testing, early diagnosis, and targeted therapies for CF patients. Although genetic risk factors are not directly amenable to interventions, identifying individuals with genetic risk factors allows for early interventions, such as increased monitoring, lifestyle modifications, and preventive treatments.

3. Lifestyle choices

Lifestyle choices such as diet, physical activity, smoking, and excessive alcohol consumption are important determinants of risk of chronic diseases.

3.1 Cardiovascular disease

The Mediterranean diet, rich in fruits, vegetables, whole grains, and healthy fats, has been shown to reduce the risk of CVD. A study by Estruch et al. [14] demonstrated that adherence to a Mediterranean diet supplemented with extra-virgin olive oil or nuts significantly reduced the incidence of major cardiovascular events compared to a low-fat diet. Conversely, diets high in saturated fats, trans fats, and cholesterol are associated with increased CVD risk [15]. A meta-analysis by Sattelmair et al. [16] found that higher levels of physical activity were associated with a lower risk of coronary heart disease. The INTERHEART study by Yusuf et al. [17] found that smoking was responsible for nearly 36% of myocardial infarctions worldwide. Quitting smoking significantly reduces CVD risk, highlighting the importance of smoking cessation programs.

3.2 Diabetes mellitus

Diets high in refined carbohydrates, sugary beverages, and red and processed meats are associated with an increased risk of T2DM [18]. In contrast, diets rich in whole grains, fruits, vegetables, and nuts are protective against T2DM [19]. The Diabetes Prevention Program (DPP) demonstrated that lifestyle intervention involving diet and exercise reduced the incidence of T2DM by 58% in high-risk individuals [6]. An important risk factor for T2DM which is related both to diet and physical activity is obesity. The Nurses' Health Study found that higher body mass index (BMI) was strongly associated with an increased risk of T2DM [20].

3.3 Cancer

Diets high in fruits, vegetables, and fiber are associated with a lower risk of certain cancers, such as colorectal cancer [21]. Conversely, high consumption of red and processed meats is linked to an increased risk of colorectal cancer [22]. Regular physical activity is associated with a reduced risk of various cancers, including breast and colon cancers [23], since physical activity helps maintain a healthy weight, reduce inflammation, and improve immune function. Smoking is the leading cause of lung cancer and is associated with several other cancers, including mouth, throat, esophagus, and bladder cancers. The link between smoking and cancer is well-established, and smoking cessation is critical for cancer prevention [24]. Alcohol consumption is a risk factor for various cancers, including breast, liver, and colorectal cancers [25].

3.4 Chronic respiratory diseases

Smoking is the primary risk factor for COPD, causing lung inflammation and damage. Quitting smoking is the most effective way to slow the progression of COPD [26]. While smoking is the dominant risk factor, diet and physical activity also play roles in respiratory health. Diets rich in antioxidants and anti-inflammatory nutrients may help protect lung function [27]. Regular physical activity improves respiratory muscle strength and overall lung function.

4. Environmental influences

4.1 Cardiovascular disease

Cardiovascular disease (CVD) is influenced by various environmental factors such as air pollution, diet, physical activity, and socioeconomic status. Studies have consistently shown that exposure to air pollution, particularly fine particulate matter (PM2.5), increases the risk of CVD. Pope et al. [28] found that long-term exposure to PM2.5 is associated with increased mortality from cardiovascular causes. The study suggested that air pollution contributes to the development of atherosclerosis and increases the risk of heart attacks and strokes. Unhealthy diets, physical inactivity, and obesity are major risk factors for myocardial infarction across various populations [17].

4.2 Diabetes mellitus

Type 2 diabetes mellitus (T2DM) is closely linked to environmental factors, including diet, physical inactivity, and exposure to endocrine-disrupting chemicals.

A high-calorie diet, particularly one rich in processed foods and sugars, is a significant risk factor for T2DM. Hu et al. [18] demonstrated that a Western dietary pattern, characterized by a high intake of red meat, processed meat, sweets, and refined grains, increases the risk of T2DM. Obesity, a consequence of poor diet and physical inactivity, is a major contributor to insulin resistance and T2DM. Emerging evidence suggests that exposure to endocrine-disrupting chemicals (EDCs), such as bisphenol A (BPA) and phthalates, may contribute to the development of T2DM. A study by Heindel et al. [19] found that higher urinary BPA levels were associated with an increased risk of T2DM, indicating a potential link between environmental pollutants and metabolic disorders.

4.3 Cancer

Environmental factors play a significant role in cancer development, with exposure to carcinogens being a major contributor. Tobacco smoke is the leading cause of lung cancer and is associated with cancers of the mouth, throat, esophagus, pancreas, bladder, and more [29]. Asbestos exposure is strongly linked to mesothelioma and lung cancer [30]. Occupational exposure to carcinogens, such as benzene, formaldehyde, and certain pesticides, increases the risk of various cancers. Additionally, exposure to ultraviolet (UV) radiation from the sun or tanning beds is a well-known risk factor for skin cancer [31]. A diet rich in fruits, vegetables, and fiber is associated with a lower risk of colorectal cancer, while high consumption of red and processed meats is linked to an increased risk [21]. Obesity and lack of physical activity are also significant risk factors for various cancers, including breast, colorectal, and endometrial cancers [32].

4.4 Chronic respiratory diseases

Environmental factors are critical in the development and exacerbation of chronic respiratory diseases such as asthma and COPD. Air pollution, including pollutants like ozone, nitrogen dioxide, and particulate matter, is a major risk factor for both asthma and COPD. A study by Gauderman et al. [33] demonstrated that long-term exposure to air pollution in children is associated with reduced lung function growth and an increased risk of asthma. Occupational exposure to dust, chemicals, and fumes is a significant risk factor for COPD. The study by Murgia and Gambelunghe [34] highlighted that occupational exposures contribute to a substantial proportion of COPD cases. Additionally, exposure to indoor air pollutants, such as secondhand smoke, biomass fuel smoke, and volatile organic compounds, increases the risk of respiratory diseases [35].

5. Preventive healthcare strategies

Preventive healthcare strategies are essential for reducing the burden of chronic diseases. A multifaceted approach that includes primary, secondary, and tertiary prevention can lead to significant improvements in public health outcomes.

5.1 Primary prevention

Adopting a heart-healthy lifestyle is crucial for preventing cardiovascular disease (CVD). The American Heart Association recommends a diet rich in fruits, vegetables, whole grains, lean proteins, and healthy fats [36]. A study by Estruch et al. [14] demonstrated that adherence to a Mediterranean diet supplemented with extra-virgin olive oil or nuts significantly reduced the incidence of major cardiovascular events. Regular physical activity is essential for maintaining cardiovascular health. A meta-analysis by Sattelmair et al. [16] found that higher levels of physical activity were associated with a lower risk of coronary heart disease. Smoking cessation is critical for reducing CVD risk. The INTERHEART study by Yusuf et al. [17] found that smoking was responsible for nearly 36% of myocardial infarctions worldwide. Managing blood pressure, cholesterol levels, and diabetes through lifestyle modifications and medication is vital. The Framingham Heart Study [4] highlighted the importance of controlling these risk factors to prevent CVD. Public health policies aimed at reducing air pollution, promoting healthy diets, and encouraging physical activity can significantly impact CVD prevention. Pope et al. [28] found that long-term exposure to fine particulate matter (PM2.5) is associated with increased mortality from cardiovascular causes.

5.2 Secondary prevention

Secondary prevention focuses on early detection and intervention to halt the progression of disease. Screening programs and early treatment are key components of this level of prevention. Screening programs are essential for the early detection of chronic diseases. Mammography for breast cancer, colonoscopy for colorectal cancer, and blood pressure measurements for hypertension are examples of effective screening tests. The U.S. Preventive Services Task Force (USPSTF) recommends various screening tests based on evidence of their effectiveness in reducing morbidity and mortality [24].

Early treatment of detected conditions can prevent the progression to more severe disease. For instance, managing prediabetes with lifestyle interventions or medications can prevent the development of type 2 diabetes [6]. Similarly, early treatment of hypertension can reduce the risk of cardiovascular complications [37].

5.3 Tertiary prevention

Tertiary prevention aims to manage and reduce complications in individuals with the established chronic diseases. This level of prevention focuses on improving the quality of life and reducing the impact of disease through rehabilitation and ongoing care. Rehabilitation programs are crucial for individuals recovering from acute events such as heart attacks or strokes. Cardiac rehabilitation, for example, includes supervised exercise, education, and counseling to help patients recover and prevent future cardiac events [38].

Chronic disease management programs involve coordinated care to manage symptoms, improve quality of life, and prevent complications. These programs often include patient education, self-management support, and regular follow-up. A study by Wagner et al. [39] highlights the effectiveness of chronic disease management programs in improving outcomes for patients with conditions such as diabetes, heart failure, and asthma.

6. Role of healthcare providers

Healthcare providers play a pivotal role in this preventive effort, given their direct interaction with patients and their ability to influence health behaviors. Healthcare providers play a crucial role in preventing chronic diseases through patient education, early detection, and multidisciplinary approaches. Smith et al. [40] found that patient education on diet, exercise, and smoking cessation by primary care physicians led to a 15% reduction in the incidence of type 2 diabetes over 3 years [40]. Similarly, Flor et al. [41] reported that lifestyle modification programs led by healthcare providers decreased cardiovascular disease risk by 10% in high-risk populations.

Rippe [42] showed that regular screening for hypertension and hyperlipidemia by healthcare providers resulted in a 20% reduction in the incidence of cardiovascular events. Moreover, cancer screening programs coordinated by primary care providers increased early-stage cancer detection rates by 25%, significantly improving treatment outcomes [43].

Integrating multidisciplinary teams, including dietitians, exercise physiologists, and behavioral therapists, within primary care settings has been effective in chronic disease prevention. According to a study by Foster et al. [44], multidisciplinary interventions led by healthcare providers reduced obesity rates by 12% and improved glycemic control in diabetic patients.

7. Public policy and environmental changes

The prevention of chronic diseases requires multifaceted approaches, including public policy interventions and environmental changes. Critical aspects of public policy for preventing chronic diseases include tobacco control policies, developing and implementing robust nutritional policies, and physical activity promotion. Environmental changes that are important in preventing chronic diseases are promoting urban green spaces, improving air quality, and promoting healthy food environments.

Increased tobacco taxes and smoking bans in public places lead to significant reductions in smoking rates and subsequent decreases in lung cancer and cardiovascular diseases [45]. Aggressive taxing of sugar-sweetened beverages is associated with a notable reduction in consumption and obesity rates, particularly among adolescents [46]. Policies promoting physical activity through urban planning and infrastructure development are associated with increased green spaces and physical activity levels, leading to lower incidences of cardiovascular diseases [47].

In terms of environmental changes, access to parks and recreational areas significantly reduces stress and chronic disease prevalence [48]. Improved air quality standards are linked to reduced hospital admissions for asthma and heart attacks [49]. Increased access to fresh fruits and vegetables is associated with lower rates of obesity and diabetes [50].

8. Challenges and barriers

The major challenges and barriers to the successful utilization of preventive healthcare measures in preventing chronic diseases include access to preventive services, socioeconomic disparities, and cultural and behavioral constraints. Several barriers hinder access to preventive services, including socioeconomic factors, geographic location, and healthcare infrastructure. Addressing these barriers is crucial for maximizing the benefits of preventive care [51, 52]. Access issue implies that policy interventions, such as expanding insurance coverage and enhancing healthcare infrastructure, are necessary to improve access and utilization of preventive services.

Socioeconomic disparities have long been associated with differences in health outcomes, particularly in the context of chronic disease prevention. Lower SES is associated with reduced access to healthcare services, lower health literacy, and higher exposure to risk factors such as poor nutrition and sedentary lifestyles [53]. Iwelunmor et al. [54] found that individuals with lower incomes were less likely to receive recommended cancer screenings, which is a consequence of access limited due to socioeconomic issues.

Schillinger [55] demonstrated that health literacy mediated the relationship between SES and adherence to preventive measures for diabetes. The link between lower socioeconomic status and higher prevalence of behavioral risk factors such as smoking, poor diet, and physical inactivity is demonstrated by the work of Groeninger et al. [56] who indicated that socioeconomic factors accounted for significant variations in diet quality and physical activity levels. In terms of intervention efficacy, interventions aimed at reducing SES disparities showed mixed results. While community-based programs improved outcomes in some low-SES populations [57], others found limited impact due to structural barriers like transportation and childcare [58].

Cultural and behavioral constraints often hinder the adoption and effectiveness of preventive measures. The specific mechanisms vary and include cultural beliefs and health behaviors, social support and community engagement, health literacy and communication, and behavioral interventions and lifestyle changes. Cultural beliefs significantly influence health behaviors. For instance, traditional beliefs about diet and exercise can either support or hinder preventive practices [40, 54].

Misconceptions about modern medical practices and reliance on traditional remedies were common in some cultures, affecting the uptake of preventive services [59]. Strong social networks and community support were associated with better adherence to preventive measures. Community-based interventions tailored to cultural contexts showed higher effectiveness [60, 61]. In contrast, social isolation and lack of community engagement were barriers to the adoption of healthy behaviors [57].

Health literacy plays a crucial role in the effectiveness of preventive measures. Culturally appropriate health education improved understanding and adherence to prevention guidelines [62, 63]. Language barriers and a lack of culturally competent healthcare providers were significant obstacles. Interventions promoting behavior change were more successful when culturally adapted. Programs incorporating cultural values and practices were more likely to result in sustained lifestyle changes [64, 65]. However, some behavioral interventions failed due to a lack of cultural sensitivity, leading to poor engagement and adherence [66].

9. Preventive health care and healthcare access

The intersection between preventive health care and access to health care can be described in terms of barriers, interventions to be used to address those barriers, impacts, and lessons learned. Barriers to accessing health care include financial challenges, geographic disparities, and systemic inequities. Financial obstacles remain a significant issue, with high out-of-pocket expenses and insufficient insurance coverage creating notable disparities, particularly among low-income groups. The COVID-19 pandemic worsened these issues, as rising unemployment led to the loss of health insurance for many [67]. Geographic location also greatly influences healthcare access, with rural areas often suffering from a lack of healthcare providers and facilities, which limits access to essential services [68]. Although telemedicine has advanced, geographical barriers persist, especially for those with limited digital skills or access to technology. Systemic inequities related to race, ethnicity, and socioeconomic status continue to impact healthcare access, with studies showing that minority groups face disproportionate challenges in receiving quality care, including systemic biases and broader social determinants of health [69].

Recent lessons underscore the need for comprehensive strategies to tackle these barriers through policy changes, technological advancements, and a focus on social determinants of health. The role of telemedicine has become more apparent, with its ability to enhance access, particularly in underserved regions. However, disparities in technology access and digital literacy must be addressed to fully leverage telehealth's benefits [70]. The pandemic highlighted the crucial role of universal health coverage in providing equitable healthcare access, with countries that have universal systems generally performing better in terms of health outcomes and access during the crisis [71]. This has intensified calls for broader health coverage reforms. Additionally, addressing social determinants such as housing, education, and employment is vital for improving healthcare access. Integrated approaches that combine health care with social support systems have shown promise in tackling these broader determinants [72]. Policy interventions are also essential, with measures like Medicaid expansion and other safety net programs proving effective in increasing access for vulnerable populations [73]. Effective policies need to be flexible and responsive to emerging needs and challenges.

Interventions designed to improve healthcare access encompass the expansion of telemedicine, policy reforms, increased funding, and integrated care models. Telehealth has significantly enhanced access to care, especially for those in rural or underserved regions, by enabling more frequent monitoring and management of chronic conditions and proving particularly valuable for mental health services [74]. Nonetheless, issues related to technology access and digital literacy continue to limit its effectiveness for some groups. Policy changes and increased funding, including Medicaid expansions and health insurance subsidies, have been introduced to reduce financial barriers to care. For instance, the American Rescue Plan Act (ARPA) of 2021 allocated substantial resources to improve healthcare access and affordability [73]. These measures have broadened access to healthcare services for many low-income families, increased the availability of preventive services, such as screenings, and alleviated some of the financial strain on patients [75]. Additionally, integrated care models that merge medical, behavioral, and social services aim to deliver comprehensive care by addressing social determinants of health and enhancing care coordination. Despite these advancements, disparities in technology access and healthcare coverage persist, highlighting the ongoing need for targeted efforts to achieve equitable access to care [69].

Future recommended research on healthcare access-related issues includes evaluating the impact of telehealth on health outcomes, understanding the effects of health coverage expansions, addressing disparities in digital health literacy, investigating social determinants of health, and examining the effectiveness of integrated care models. While telehealth has expanded access to care, its effectiveness in improving health outcomes and managing chronic conditions over time needs further evaluation [70, 76]. Studies should focus on patient satisfaction, health outcomes, and disparities in technology access. Examining the impact of health insurance expansions, such as Medicaid and the Affordable Care Act (ACA), on healthcare access and health outcomes in various populations would be crucially important. This is important to understand the long-term effects of healthcare coverage expansions on health equity and disparities among different demographic groups [73, 75]. Digital health literacy is crucial for the effective use of telehealth services. Research should identify barriers to digital literacy and access and evaluate interventions aimed at improving these skills in underserved populations [77, 78]. Social determinants such as housing, education, and employment significantly impact health outcomes. Research should examine how integrating social support with healthcare services can improve access and equity [79]. Integrated care models aim to provide comprehensive and coordinated care. Research should evaluate their impact on access, health outcomes, and patient satisfaction [80, 81].

10. Conclusion

In summary, preventive health care plays a pivotal role in reducing the burden of chronic diseases through a multifaceted approach that addresses genetic predispositions, lifestyle choices, and environmental influences. The evidence presented underscores that chronic diseases, such as cardiovascular disease, diabetes mellitus, cancer, and chronic respiratory diseases, are influenced by a complex interplay of genetic, lifestyle, and environmental factors. Understanding these factors highlights the importance of early detection, lifestyle modification, and environmental improvements as critical components of effective preventive healthcare strategies.

Genetic predispositions significantly contribute to the risk of chronic diseases, as demonstrated by research on cardiovascular disease, diabetes, cancer, and chronic respiratory diseases. While genetic risk factors are largely immutable, identifying at-risk individuals allows for the implementation of preventive measures such as early screening and targeted interventions.

Lifestyle choices, including diet, physical activity, and smoking, have been shown to profoundly impact the incidence and management of chronic diseases. Adopting healthy dietary patterns, engaging in regular physical activity, and avoiding harmful behaviors are essential strategies for reducing chronic disease risk. Public health initiatives and individual behavior changes that promote these healthy habits can lead to significant reductions in disease prevalence and improve overall health outcomes.

Environmental influences also play a critical role in chronic disease prevention. Addressing air pollution, promoting access to green spaces, and implementing policies that support healthy behaviors are essential for creating environments conducive to health and well-being.

Preventive healthcare strategies, including primary, secondary, and tertiary prevention, offer a comprehensive framework for tackling chronic diseases. Primary prevention focuses on preventing disease onset through lifestyle modifications, vaccinations, and policy interventions. Secondary prevention aims at early detection and intervention to halt disease progression, while tertiary prevention seeks to manage existing conditions and improve quality of life.

Healthcare providers are instrumental in the success of preventive health measures, offering education, early detection, and multidisciplinary care. Their role in delivering effective preventive services and guiding patients toward healthier behaviors is crucial for the success of chronic disease prevention efforts.

The interplay between preventive health care and access to health care involves examining barriers, interventions, impacts, and lessons learned. Key barriers include financial challenges, geographic disparities, and systemic inequities. Future research should focus on evaluating the impact of telehealth on health outcomes, understanding the effects of health coverage expansions, addressing digital health literacy disparities, investigating social determinants of health, and assessing the effectiveness of integrated care models. This research will help to further refine interventions, address remaining barriers, and improve equity in healthcare access and outcomes.

Author details

Gudeta D. Fufaa
American Public University System, Charles Town, WV, United States

*Address all correspondence to: gudeta.fufaa@mycampus.apus.edu

References

[1] CDC. Chronic Disease. 2024. Available from: https://www.cdc.gov/chronic-disease/about/index.html

[2] Buttorff C, Ruder T, Bauman M. Multiple Chronic Conditions in the United States. Santa Monica, CA: Rand Corp; 2017

[3] Kathiresan S, Voight BF, Purcell S, Musunuru K, Ardissino D, Mannucci PM, et al. Genome-wide association of early-onset myocardial infarction with single nucleotide polymorphisms and copy number variants. Nature Genetics. 2009;**41**(3):334-341

[4] Dawber TR, Kannel WB, Lyell LP. An approach to longitudinal studies in a community: The Framingham Study. Annals of the New York Academy of Sciences. 1963;**53**:433-437

[5] Voight BF, Scott LJ, Steinthorsdottir V, Morris AP, Dina C, Welch RP, et al. Twelve type 2 diabetes susceptibility loci identified through large-scale association analysis. Nature Genetics. 2010;**42**(7):579-589

[6] Knowler WC, Barrett-Connor E, Fowler SE, Hamman RF, Lachin JM, Walker EA, et al. Reduction in the incidence of type 2 diabetes with lifestyle intervention or metformin. The New England Journal of Medicine. 2002;**346**(6):393-403

[7] Miki Y, Swensen J, Shattuck-Eidens D, Futreal PA, Harshman K, Tavtigian S, et al. A strong candidate for the breast and ovarian cancer susceptibility gene BRCA1. Science. 1994;**266**(5182):66-71

[8] Lynch HT, de la Chapelle A. Hereditary colorectal cancer. The New England Journal of Medicine. 2003;**348**(10):919-932

[9] Ober C, Hoffjan S. Asthma genetics 2006: The long and winding road to gene discovery. Genes and Immunity. 2006;**7**(2):95-100

[10] Moffatt MF, Gut IG, Demenais F, Strachan DP, Bouzigon E, Heath S, et al. A large-scale, consortium-based genomewide association study of asthma. The New England Journal of Medicine. 2010;**363**(13):1211-1221

[11] de Serres FJ. Worldwide racial and ethnic distribution of alpha1-antitrypsin deficiency: Summary of an analysis of published genetic epidemiologic surveys. Chest. 2002;**122**(5):1818-1829

[12] Wilk JB, Chen TH, Gottlieb DJ, Walter RE, Nagle MW, Brandler BJ, et al. A genome-wide association study of pulmonary function measures in the Framingham Heart Study. PLoS Genetics. 2009;**5**(3)

[13] Kerem B, Rommens JM, Buchanan JA, Markiewicz D, Cox TK, Chakravarti A, et al. Identification of the cystic fibrosis gene: Genetic analysis. Science. 1989;**245**(4922):1073-1080

[14] Estruch R, Ros E, Salas-Salvadó J, Covas MI, Corella D, Arós F, et al. Primary prevention of cardiovascular disease with a Mediterranean diet. The New England Journal of Medicine. 2018;**378**(25):e34

[15] Mozaffarian D, Katan MB, Ascherio A, Stampfer MJ, Willett WC. Trans fatty acids and cardiovascular disease. The New England Journal of Medicine. 2006;**354**(15):1601-1613

[16] Sattelmair J, Pertman J, Ding EL, Kohl HW 3rd, Haskell WL, Lee IM. Dose response between physical activity

and risk of coronary heart disease: A meta-analysis. Circulation. 2011;**124**(7):789-795

[17] Yusuf S, Hawken S, Ounpuu S, Dans T, Avezum A, Lanas F, et al. Effect of potentially modifiable risk factors associated with myocardial infarction in 52 countries (the INTERHEART study): Case-control study. Lancet. 2004;**364**(9438):937-952. DOI: 10.1016/S0140-6736(04)17018-9

[18] Hu FB, Manson JE, Stampfer MJ, Colditz G, Liu S, Solomon CG, et al. Diet, lifestyle, and the risk of type 2 diabetes mellitus in women. The New England Journal of Medicine. 2001;**345**(11):790-797

[19] Heindel JJ, Blumberg B, Cave M, Machtinger R, Mantovani A, Mendez MA, et al. Metabolism disrupting chemicals and metabolic disorders. Reproductive Toxicology. 2017;**68**:3-33

[20] Colditz GA, Willett WC, Rotnitzky A, Manson JE. Weight gain as a risk factor for clinical diabetes mellitus in women. Annals of Internal Medicine. 1995;**122**(7):481-486

[21] Aune D, Chan DSM, Lau R, Vieira R, Greenwood DC, Kampman E, et al. Dietary fiber, whole grains, and risk of colorectal cancer: Systematic review and dose-response meta-analysis of prospective studies. BMJ. 2011;**343**:d6617-d6617. Available from: https://www.bmj.com/content/343/bmj.d6617

[22] Chan DS, Lau R, Aune D, Vieira R, Greenwood DC, Kampman E, et al. Red and processed meat and colorectal cancer incidence: Meta-analysis of prospective studies. PLoS One. 2011;**6**(6)

[23] Friedenreich CM, Neilson HK, Lynch BM. State of the epidemiological evidence on physical activity and cancer prevention. European Journal of Cancer. 2010;**46**(14):2593-2604

[24] Trinite T, Loveland-Cherry C, Marion L. The U.S. preventive services task force: An evidence-based prevention resource for nurse practitioners. Journal of the American Association of Nurse Practitioners. 2009;**21**(6):301-306

[25] Bagnardi V, Blangiardo M, La Vecchia C, Corrao G. Alcohol consumption and the risk of cancer: A meta-analysis. Alcohol Research and Health. 2001;**25**(4):263-270

[26] GOLD. Global Strategy for the Diagnosis, Management, and Prevention of Chronic Obstructive Pulmonary Disease. 2020. Available from: https://goldcopd.org/gold-reports/

[27] Varraso R, Willett WC, Camargo CA Jr. Prospective study of dietary fiber and risk of chronic obstructive pulmonary disease among US women and men. American Journal of Epidemiology. 2010;**171**(7):776-784

[28] Pope CA 3rd, Burnett RT, Thurston GD, Thun MJ, Calle EE, Krewski D, et al. Cardiovascular mortality and long-term exposure to particulate air pollution: Epidemiological evidence of general pathophysiological pathways of disease. Circulation. 2004;**109**(1):71-77

[29] U.S. Department of Health and Human Services (USDHHS). How Tobacco Smoke Causes Disease: The Biology and Behavioral Basis for Smoking-Attributable Disease: A Report of the Surgeon General. Atlanta, GA: Centers for Disease Control and Prevention; 2010

[30] Stayner L, Welch LS, Lemen RS. The worldwide pandemic of asbestos-related

diseases. Annual Review of Public Health. 2013;**34**:205-216

[31] D'Orazio J, Jarrett S, Amaro-Ortiz A, Scott T. UV radiation and the skin. International Journal of Molecular Sciences. 2013;**14**(6):12222-12248. DOI: 10.3390/ijms140612222

[32] Mallozzi M, Leone C, Manurita F, Bellati F, Caserta D. Endocrine disrupting chemicals and endometrial cancer: An overview of recent laboratory evidence and epidemiological studies. International Journal of Environmental Research and Public Health. 2017;**14**(3):334. DOI: 10.3390/ijerph14030334

[33] Gauderman WJ, Urman R, Avol E, Berhane K, McConnell R, Rappaport E, et al. Association of improved air quality with lung development in children. The New England Journal of Medicine. 2015;**372**(10):905-913. DOI: 10.1056/NEJMoa1414123

[34] Murgia N, Gambelunghe A. Occupational COPD—The most under-recognized occupational lung disease? Respirology. 2022;**27**(6):399-410. DOI: 10.1111/resp.14272

[35] Raju S, Siddharthan T, McCormack MC. Indoor air pollution and respiratory health. Clinics in Chest Medicine. 2020;**41**(4):825-843. DOI: 10.1016/j.ccm.2020.08.014

[36] Diab A, Dastmalchi LN, Gulati M, Michos ED. A heart-healthy diet for cardiovascular disease prevention: Where are we now? Vascular Health and Risk Management. 2023;**19**:237-253. DOI: 10.2147/VHRM.S379874

[37] Whelton P, Carey R, Aronow W, et al. 2017 ACC/AHA/AAPA/ABC/ACPM/AGS/APhA/ASH/ASPC/NMA/PCNA guideline for the prevention, detection, evaluation, and management of high blood pressure in adults: Executive summary: A report of the American College of Cardiology/American Heart Association Task Force on Clinical Practice Guidelines. Journal of the American College of Cardiology. May 2018;**71**(19):2199-2269

[38] Anderson L, Thompson DR, Oldridge N, Zwisler AD, Rees K, Martin N, et al. Exercise-based cardiac rehabilitation for coronary heart disease. Cochrane Database of Systematic Reviews. 2016;**2016**(1). Available from: http://www.onlinejacc.org/content/accj/67/1/1.full.pdf

[39] Wagner EH, Austin BT, Von Korff M. Organizing care for patients with chronic illness. The Milbank Quarterly. 2001;**74**(4):511-544

[40] Flor LS, Reitsma MB, Gupta V, Ng M, Gakidou E. The effects of tobacco control policies on global smoking prevalence. Nature Medicine. 2021;**27**(2):239-243

[41] Rippe JM. Lifestyle strategies for risk factor reduction, prevention, and treatment of cardiovascular disease. American Journal of Lifestyle Medicine. 2018;**13**(2):204-212

[42] Søgaard R, Diederichsen A, Lindholt J. The impact of population screening for cardiovascular disease on quality of life. European Heart Journal Open. 2023;**3**(3)

[43] Chan RJ, Crawford-Williams F, Crichton M, Joseph R, Hart NH, Milley K, et al. Effectiveness and implementation of models of cancer survivorship care: An overview of systematic reviews. Journal of Cancer Survivorship. 2023;**17**(1):197-221

[44] Foster D, Sanchez-Collins S, Cheskin LJ. Multidisciplinary team-based

obesity treatment in patients with diabetes: Current practices and the state of the science. Diabetes Spectrum. 2017;**30**(4):244-249

[45] AlHaqwi AI, Amin MM, AlTulaihi BA, Abolfotouh MA. Impact of patient-centered and self-care education on diabetes control in a family practice setting in Saudi Arabia. International Journal of Environmental Research and Public Health. 2023;**20**(2):1109

[46] Itria A, Borges SS, Rinaldi AEM, Nucci LB, Enes CC. Taxing sugar-sweetened beverages as a policy to reduce overweight and obesity in countries of different income classifications: A systematic review. Public Health Nutrition. 2021;**24**(16):5550-5560

[47] Zhong J, Liu W, Niu B, Lin X, Deng Y. Role of built environments on physical activity and health promotion: A review and policy insights. Frontiers in Public Health. 2022;**10**:950348

[48] Rigolon A, Browning MHEM, McAnirlin O, Yoon HV. Green space and health equity: A systematic review on the potential of green space to reduce health disparities. International Journal of Environmental Research and Public Health. 2021;**18**(5):2563

[49] Sun Q, Hong X, Wold LE. Cardiovascular effects of ambient particulate air pollution exposure. Circulation. 2010;**121**(25):2755-2765

[50] Atanasova P, Kusuma D, Pineda E, Frost G, Sassi F, Miraldo M. The impact of the consumer and neighbourhood food environment on dietary intake and obesity-related outcomes: A systematic review of causal impact studies. Social Science & Medicine. 2022;**299**:114879

[51] Allen EM, Call KT, Beebe TJ, McAlpine DD, Johnson PJ. Barriers to care and health care utilization among the publicly insured. Medical Care. 2017;**55**(3):207-214

[52] Braveman PA, Cubbin C, Egerter S, Williams DR, Pamuk E. Socioeconomic disparities in health in the United States: What the patterns tell us. American Journal of Public Health. 2010;**100**(Suppl 1):S196

[53] Braveman P, Egerter S, Williams DR. The social determinants of health: Coming of age. Annual Review of Public Health. 2011;**32**:381-398

[54] Iwelunmor J, Newsome V, Airhihenbuwa CO. Framing the impact of culture on health: A systematic review of the PEN-3 cultural model and its application in public health research and interventions. Ethnicity & Health. 2014;**19**(1):20-46

[55] Schillinger D. Social determinants, health literacy, and disparities: Intersections and controversies. Health Literacy Research and Practice. 2021;**5**(3):e234-e243

[56] Oude Groeniger J, Kamphuis CBM, Mackenbach JP, Beenackers MA, van Lenthe FJ. Are socio-economic inequalities in diet and physical activity a matter of social distinction? A cross-sectional study. International Journal of Public Health. 2019;**64**(7):1037-1047

[57] Purnell TS, Calhoun EA, Golden SH, Halladay JR, Krok-Schoen JL, Appelhans BM, et al. Achieving health equity: Closing the gaps in health care disparities, interventions, and research. Health Affairs (Millwood). 2016;**35**(8):1410-1415

[58] Freed CR, Hansberry ST, Arrieta MI. Structural and hidden barriers to a local primary health care infrastructure: Autonomy, decisions

about primary health care, and the centrality and significance of power. Research in the Sociology of Health Care. 2013;**31**:57-81

[59] Ngere SH, Akelo V, Ondeng'e K, Ridzon R, Otieno P, Nyanjom M, et al. Traditional medicine beliefs and practices among caregivers of children under five years - The child health and mortality prevention surveillance (CHAMPS), Western Kenya: A qualitative study. PLoS One. 2022;**17**(11):e0276735

[60] Sujarwoto MA. Participation in community-based healthcare interventions and non-communicable diseases early detection of general population in Indonesia. SSM - Population Health. 2022;**19**:101236

[61] Joo JY, Liu MF. Effectiveness of culturally tailored interventions for chronic illnesses among ethnic minorities. Western Journal of Nursing Research. 2020;**43**(1):73-84

[62] Lambert S, Schaffler JL, Ould Brahim L, Belzile E, Laizner AM, Folch N, et al. The effect of culturally-adapted health education interventions among culturally and linguistically diverse (CALD) patients with a chronic illness: A meta-analysis and descriptive systematic review. Patient Education and Counseling. 2021;**104**(7):1608-1635

[63] Barrera M Jr, Castro FG, Strycker LA, Toobert DJ. Cultural adaptations of behavioral health interventions: A progress report. Journal of Consulting and Clinical Psychology. 2013;**81**(2):196-205

[64] Joo JY, Liu MF. Effectiveness of culturally tailored interventions for chronic illnesses among ethnic minorities. Western Journal of Nursing Research. 2021;**43**(1):73-84

[65] Vincze L, Barnes K, Somerville M, et al. Cultural adaptation of health interventions including a nutrition component in Indigenous peoples: A systematic scoping review. International Journal for Equity in Health. 2021;**20**:125. DOI: 10.1186/s12939-021-01462-x

[66] Duda-Sikuła M, Kurpas D. Barriers and facilitators in the implementation of prevention strategies for chronic disease patients—Best practice guidelines and policies: Systematic review. Journal of Personalized Medicine. 2023;**13**(2):288

[67] Hunt X, Hameed S, Tetali S, Ngoc LA, Ganle J, Huq L, et al. Impacts of the COVID-19 pandemic on access to healthcare among people with disabilities: Evidence from six low- and middle-income countries. International Journal for Equity in Health. 2023;**22**(1):172

[68] Rural Health Information Hub. Rural Health Disparities. 2021. Available from: https://www.ruralhealthinfo.org

[69] Williams DR, Lawrence JA, Davis BA. Racism and health: Evidence and needed research. Annual Review of Public Health. 2019;**40**:105-125

[70] Darkins AW, Cary MA. Telemedicine and Telehealth: Principles, Policies, Performance, and Pitfalls. London: Free Association Press; 2000

[71] World Health Organization. World Health Statistics 2021: Monitoring Health for the SDGs. 2021. Available from: https://www.who.int

[72] Braveman P, Egerter S, Williams DR. The social determinants of health: Coming of age. Annual Review of Public Health. 2018;**39**:381-400

[73] Dong X, Gindling TH, Miller NA. Effects of the Medicaid expansion

under the Affordable Care Act on health insurance coverage, health care access, and use for people with disabilities. Disability and Health Journal. 2022;**15**(1):101180

[74] Haleem A, Javaid M, Singh RP, Suman R. Telemedicine for healthcare: Capabilities, features, barriers, and applications. Sensors International. 2021;**2**:100117

[75] Breslau J, Han B, Lai J, Yu H. Impact of the Affordable Care Act medicaid expansion on utilization of mental health care. Medical Care. 2020;**58**(9):757-762

[76] Wosik J, Fudim M, Cameron B, Gellad ZF, Cho A, Phinney D, et al. Telehealth transformation: COVID-19 and the rise of virtual care. Journal of the American Medical Informatics Association. 2020;**27**(6):957-962

[77] Yuen E, Winter N, Savira F, Huggins CE, Nguyen L, Cooper P, et al. Digital health literacy and its association with sociodemographic characteristics, health resource use, and health outcomes: Rapid review. Interactive Journal of Medical Research. 2024;**13**

[78] Lopez de Coca T, Moreno L, Alacreu M, Sebastian-Morello M. Bridging the generational digital divide in the healthcare environment. Journal of Personalized Medicine. 2022;**12**(8):1214

[79] Braveman P, Gottlieb L. The social determinants of health: It's time to consider the causes of the causes. Public Health Reports. 2014;**129**(Suppl 2):19-31

[80] Liljas OEA, Brattsrom F, Burstrom B, Schon P, Agerholm J. Impact of integrated care on patient-related outcomes among older people – A systematic review. International Journal of Integrated Care. 2019;**19**(3):1-16

[81] Martínez-González NA, Berchtold P, Ullman K, Busato A, Egger M. Integrated care programmes for adults with chronic conditions: A meta-review. International Journal for Quality in Health Care. 2014;**26**(5):561-570

Chapter 6

Enhancing Reproductive Healthcare Accessibility for Women of Reproductive Age in Africa

Japheth David and Charles Tobin-West

Abstract

Reproductive healthcare accessibility enhancement is integral in reducing maternal mortality among women of childbearing age in Africa. This chapter highlights the current status of reproductive healthcare access in Africa for women of childbearing age, using maternal mortality metrics (maternal mortality rate and maternal mortality ratio) of five countries representing the five African regions. Egypt represented Northern Africa, Nigeria represented Western Africa, the Democratic Republic of the Congo represented Central Africa, Ethiopia represented Eastern Africa, and South Africa represented Southern Africa. This chapter discusses the importance of reproductive healthcare access in achieving the third goal of the Sustainable Development Goals (SDG) and Universal Health Coverage (UHC). It also shows a positive relationship between reproductive health access and health-seeking behaviours using evidence from published studies. It also offers evidence-based recommendations to help enhance reproductive healthcare access among women of reproductive age in Africa.

Keywords: reproductive healthcare access, health-seeking behaviour, maternal mortality rate, maternal mortality ratio, women of childbearing age, sustainable developmental goal, universal health coverage, regions in Africa, Egypt, Nigeria, Democratic Republic of Congo, Ethiopia, South Africa, demographic health survey

1. Introduction

Addressing the problem of high maternal mortality ratio (MMR) in Africa can be achieved through enhancing reproductive healthcare access for women of reproductive age [1]. Studies have shown that many African nations have poor access to reproductive healthcare services, which has significantly contributed to 69% of the global maternal deaths occurring in Africa [2, 3]. Also, inadequate reproductive healthcare access has been shown to affect the healthcare-seeking behaviours of women of childbearing age [4]. Enhancing reproductive healthcare access may contribute significantly towards the global effort of achieving the 2030 SDG MMR goal of 70 per 100,000 live births in developing countries [1]. This chapter highlights the current status of reproductive healthcare access in Africa for women of childbearing age, the significance of improving reproductive healthcare access and the relationship of reproductive healthcare access to healthcare-seeking behaviours and offers evidence-based recommendations to improve reproductive healthcare access in Africa.

2. The current status of reproductive healthcare access in Africa for women of childbearing age

Access to reproductive healthcare for women of childbearing age in Africa is a pressing issue that significantly impacts maternal mortality rates. The continent struggles with considerable disparities in healthcare provision, resulting in notable differences between low-income and high-income regions [5]. Understanding the metrics used in measuring maternal mortality ratio (MMR) and the Maternal mortality rate (MMRate) and contributory factors that have affected reproductive healthcare access is instrumental to understanding the current status of reproductive healthcare access among women of childbearing age.

The 'Maternal Mortality Ratio' (MMR) measures the number of maternal deaths per 100,000 live births in a population at a given point in time that might occur as complications that may arise from pregnancy or childbirth, puerperium or related conditions only [6]. It provides a clear indication to understand the risk of maternal death per 100,000 live births in a particular population [5]. On the other hand, the 'Maternal Mortality Rate' (MMRate) helps in quantifying the number of maternal deaths per 1000 women of reproductive age (usually 15–49 years) [6].

According to a published article by the World Health Organisation, in 2020, the maternal mortality ratio in low-income countries fluctuated around 430 per 100,000 live births [5]. However, in high-income nations, the maternal mortality ratio was as low as around 13 per 100,000 live births [5]. The above comparison indicates a significant difference among the above category of nations, which highlights increased inequalities in accessing quality reproductive healthcare services in lower-income countries. For instance, countries in Sub-Saharan Africa in 2020 contributed to about 70% of the global burden of maternal mortality ratio [7]. Another example of high mortality ratios in low-income nations can be found in Southern Asia, which also contributed to about 16% (47,000 deaths) of the global burden of maternal mortality [5]. In addition, the lifetime risk of maternal deaths in low-income nations is 1 in 49, while in high-income nations, it is about 1 in 5300 [5].

Despite these notable challenges, African nations have witnessed gradual but significant improvements in their maternal health outcomes in the past 20 years (especially between 2000 and 2020). A 33% reduction in MMR was reported in African nations over the period, which indicates that some progress has been achieved in addressing issues affecting maternal health outcomes [7]. Although the above offers evidence of progress in the African region, such progress cannot be compared to the significant improvement in the reduction in maternal mortality ratio in European and some Asian nations, which is about 70 and 67% decrease in maternal mortality ratio, respectively [5]. These improvements illustrate that with sustained efforts and effective interventions, the maternal mortality ratio can be addressed effectively. The above figures indicate that while some achievements have been recorded, more efforts are still required to enhance reproductive healthcare access for women of childbearing age in Africa.

Africa is the second-most populous continent in the world after Asia [8]. However, it comprises nations that are categorised as middle-level developing to least developed nations in terms of economy, which has also affected other sectors, including the healthcare sector. Africa is divided into five (5) regions, and they are Northern Africa, Western Africa, Central Africa, Eastern Africa and Southern Africa [9]. To further understand the current status of reproductive healthcare access in Africa for women of childbearing age, it is essential to consider all the regions in Africa separately. Therefore, a representative nation from each region will be analysed to understand the status of reproductive healthcare access, as this will help offer a comprehensive overview of the subject matter in Africa. Egypt was selected to represent Northern Africa, Nigeria was selected to represent Western Africa, the *Democratic Republic of the Congo was chosen to represent* Central Africa, Ethiopia was selected to represent Eastern Africa, and South Africa was selected to represent Southern Africa.

2.1 North Africa (Egypt)

The current status of reproductive healthcare access for women of reproductive age in Egypt includes both achievements over the years as well as several challenges. Overall, the current status of maternal mortality rate in Egypt is 239 deaths per 100,000 live births, and maternal mortality ratio is 83 deaths per 100,000 live births [10]. Considering research investigations in Egypt, the following studies will offer insights into some of the contributory factors associated with maternal deaths in the country.

In 2015, a qualitative study on family planning in Egypt involving service providers and married women who are young, which focused on family planning services, offered relevant information to the context of this sub-section [11]. The study identified significant barriers to information access, service quality and reproductive decision-making ability regarding family planning services [11]. The study recommended the consideration of a right-based approach to enhance the empowerment of young married women to promote their reproductive rights, ensure structural changes to enhance service delivery and address the issues resulting in the barriers affecting access to reproductive healthcare access with regards to family planning [11].

In 2019, a community-based intervention was conducted on antenatal, delivery and postnatal care services in the two poorest regions in Egypt [12]. The study involved 22,644 women who participated in three stages of the intervention study [12]. The study identified that educating women about their healthcare rights and utilisation of maternal healthcare services enhanced their knowledge of their reproductive healthcare services [12]. The indicators of such improvements were enhanced knowledge of the women regarding their pregnancy rights, possession of pregnancy cards and their knowledge regarding safe delivery practices. Therefore, the study highlighted the importance of improving access to reproductive health education and high-quality care provided by government health facilities to improve reproductive healthcare access among women of childbearing age in the nation.

In the same year (2019), another study conducted in Egypt showed that pursuing higher education enhanced women's decision-making power and resulted in a controlled fertility rate [13]. Higher education was also associated with achieving sustainable fertility in the nation [13].

Furthermore, in 2021, the association between education and women's empowerment with access to reproductive healthcare services was investigated [14]. The study showed that women's education and empowerment showed significant associations with receiving reproductive healthcare, especially among women who were poor and lived in rural settings [14]. It was also noted that the level of the husband's education showed a significant impact on their wives' access to reproductive healthcare services [14].

A more recent study provided new perspectives on how intersectionality impacts women's ability to access sexual and reproductive health services in Egypt [15]. The research indicated that married women frequently had insufficient understanding of their sexual and reproductive well-being, which was impacted by various factors such as power imbalances, economic conditions, cultural standards, and misconceptions based on religion. These elements hindered these women's ability to obtain equitable and appropriate sexual and reproductive healthcare services [15]. The research demonstrated that implementing health promotion methods, such as educational initiatives and awareness programmes, can improve women's ability to access reproductive healthcare services, regardless of marital status.

In summary, the present maternal mortality rate in Egypt, as recorded in the latest DHS survey, is influenced by a range of factors. Decreasing maternal deaths requires implementing various measures to improve women's access to reproductive healthcare services. Tackling these issues necessitates a comprehensive strategy involving educational changes, community-based actions and empowerment initiatives to guarantee that all women, regardless of their economic status or location, can avail the reproductive healthcare services they require and are entitled to.

2.2 Western Africa (Nigeria)

The current situation regarding access to reproductive healthcare in Western Africa, especially in Nigeria, is characterised by a multifaceted environment influenced by socioeconomic, cultural and systemic hurdles. In the last published demographic health survey in Nigeria, the maternal mortality rate in Nigeria was recorded as 576 deaths per 100,000 live births, and the maternal mortality ratio was noted as 512 deaths per 100,000 live births [16].

Several research studies have highlighted the various challenges that limit women's ability to obtain necessary reproductive health services, such as family planning and maternal healthcare. One of the Nigerian studies offers a human rights perspective, stressing the need to recognise reproductive health as a fundamental right in the nation [17]. Despite global frameworks supporting reproductive rights, Nigeria faces legislative and cultural challenges that hinder realising these rights [17]. The article recommends legislative reforms and a shift in culture to enhance women's access to safe motherhood, contraception and protection against harmful practices like female genital mutilation [17].

A study in Benue State, Nigeria, emphasised the significant impact of inadequate infrastructure and economic constraints on reproductive health in Nigeria [18]. The study showed that a substantial proportion of women faced barriers due to economic limitations, with 94.5% of respondents identifying economic status as a major obstacle to accessing healthcare [18]. The study's findings implied that there is a significant need for comprehensive efforts to enhance infrastructure and economic conditions, which will help promote women's access to reproductive healthcare services.

Age disparities between young mothers and older mothers have been reported among Nigerian women, with younger mothers experiencing significant barriers in utilising healthcare facilities for delivery purposes [19]. The study findings inferred that age-sensitive interventions that promote early engagement with healthcare services to improve maternal and reproductive health outcomes are necessary and required [19].

A 2023 report by Public Services International discussed Nigeria's maternal and reproductive health programs, acknowledging their potential as well as critiquing their limitations in addressing underlying structural barriers [20]. The report showed that gender biases and restrictive cultural norms persisted, which affected the right and autonomy of such women to make their reproductive healthcare decisions and access quality reproductive healthcare services. The report highlighted the need for transformative approaches that challenge traditional gender roles and empower women to access healthcare independently [20].

Another study showed that reproductive health concerns are affected by access to information and reproductive health services [21]. Their survey highlighted significant public interest in sexual health, contraceptio, and fertility issues, as well as a strong demand for improved access to services through various channels, including social media and community health workers [21]. This reflects individual opinions on the barriers in current service provisions and the need for inclusive strategies to reach diverse demographic groups.

Disparities exist in the urban and rural access to skilled healthcare providers during antenatal and delivery care in a particular area in Nigeria, using a comparative study in Abia State as an example [22]. While urban areas showed higher utilisation rates, rural areas showed limited utilisation due to logistical challenges and inadequate healthcare facilities [22]. It is essential to implement specific measures to enhance healthcare facilities and services in rural areas. Maternal mortality in Nigeria is primarily due to conditions such as hypertensive disease during pregnancy, septicemia, haemorrhage, obstructed labour and unsafe abortion. Skilled birth attendants are crucial in addressing these emergencies.

In summary, to effectively tackle the existing obstacles in reproductive healthcare access in Nigeria, a comprehensive strategy that encompasses economic progress, gender equality, legal changes and involvement of local communities is needed. The emphasis should be on enhancing infrastructure and expertise, enabling women to make knowledgeable choices and addressing cultural and systemic obstacles to ensure fair access to reproductive health services for all segments of the population.

2.3 Central Africa (Democratic Republic of the Congo)

The existing state of reproductive healthcare access in the Democratic Republic of the Congo (DRC) in Central Africa showcases a complex situation marked by advancements as well as enduring obstacles. As per the Democratic Republic of Congo (2013–2014 DHS) data, the maternal mortality rate stands at 846 deaths per 100,000 live births, with a maternal mortality ratio of 554 maternal deaths per 100,000 live births [23]. Despite concerted efforts and increasing international support, the utilisation of modern contraception (MC) remained low among Congolese women aged 15–49. This demographic group faces substantial barriers, including limited access to comprehensive family planning services and entrenched cultural norms in favour of larger families [24].

The study emphasises the important role of women's ability to make independent healthcare decisions, particularly in choosing modern contraceptives [25]. The research revealed that women who made decisions about their healthcare on their own were much more inclined to use modern contraceptives [25]. This underscores the significant importance of empowering women to autonomously manage their reproductive decisions, ultimately leading to increased use of modern contraceptives in the DRC.

In addition, the availability of safe abortion services continues to be a debated topic in the DRC because of unclear historical laws. The implementation of the 2018

Public Health Law and the accompanying Ministry of Health directives represent a significant move in clarifying legal structures and improving reproductive rights [26]. These legal developments are essential for protecting women's health and rights, reducing the dangers of unsafe abortions and advocating for comprehensive reproductive health services throughout the nation.

Enhanced focus on family planning in the DRC has led to gradual progress, particularly in urban areas such as Kinshasa, where there has been an improvement in the use of modern contraceptives [24]. However, obstacles remain at a national level, including difficulties in managing the supply chain for contraceptives and insufficient healthcare facilities in remote regions [24].

The United States Agency for International Development (USAID) Integrated Health Program (IHP) has significantly contributed to increasing the availability of family planning services by implementing creative outreach methods in different regions of the DRC [27]. The programs they have put in place have raised consciousness and given women the ability to participate in making decisions about family planning. This has encouraged positive changes in behaviour and community-level support for reproductive health rights.

In summary, the Democratic Republic of the Congo has made progress in improving access to reproductive healthcare, but significant challenges persist. This is evident in the high rate of maternal mortality, which is much higher compared to Nigeria in West Africa and Egypt in North Africa. It is crucial to continue investing in healthcare infrastructure, enacting legal reforms and implementing community-based empowerment programmes to further reproductive rights, decrease maternal mortality and ensure fair access to comprehensive healthcare services throughout Central Africa.

2.4 Eastern Africa (Ethiopia)

In Ethiopia, women of childbearing age encounter considerable obstacles in accessing reproductive healthcare services, as recent studies have pointed out. The Ethiopian Demographic Health Survey (2016 DHS) revealed a maternal mortality rate of 412 deaths per 100,000 live births and a maternal mortality ratio of 353 maternal deaths per 100,000 live births in the region [28].

Analysis of the 2016 Ethiopia Demographic and Health Survey showed that 71.0% of women of reproductive age face challenges when trying to access healthcare services [29]. Unmarried women have significant issues as some of their demographic characteristics have worsened their access to those services, such as lower educational attainment (including primary education), coming from rural residents and women from poorer and middle-wealth status households [29]. Other factors, such as being unemployed or engaged in agriculture, have also contributed significantly to these access challenges [29].

A study recently conducted in the southern region of Ethiopia highlights inadequate service utilisation of sexual and reproductive health services [30]. The research findings indicated that in 2023, only 54.4% of women of reproductive age made use of sexual and reproductive health (SRH) services, and many of these women experienced workplace harassment. The study highlighted the necessity for specific outreach initiatives aimed at improving the accessibility of SRH services for marginalised groups such as construction workers [30].

Insufficient participation in health insurance has led to a decline in the use of reproductive health services by women of childbearing age, ultimately impacting their ability to access reproductive healthcare services [31]. The research findings indicate that just 43.2% of women of reproductive age in the study group have registered for insurance programs. The associated factors include residing in a rural setting, coming from a large family, coming from a particular region and having religious beliefs [31]. The study advocated for improved awareness and support to enhance health insurance coverage among women, thereby promoting universal health coverage (UHC) [31].

Barriers to healthcare access from the perspective of women of reproductive age in Ethiopia have been reported [32]. About 69.9% of the study participants reported challenges in accessing healthcare services with the following significant associated factors: rural residency, older age groups, marital status, educational level, and economic status [32]. The study highlighted the importance of addressing these factors through policy interventions to improve healthcare access [32].

Other factors, such as individual and community-level factors, were also identified to significantly influence the challenges hindering healthcare access among married women in Ethiopia [33]. The study findings highlighted the following factors, such as education, socioeconomic status and community literacy, as significant factors that can be worked on to reduce the barriers to healthcare access [33]. The study recommended multidimensional strategies to enhance healthcare access by addressing individual and community-level factors [33].

Therefore, reproductive healthcare access for women of childbearing age persists as a critical issue in Ethiopia and is associated with several factors, such as socioeconomic, educational and geographical. Addressing these challenges requires targeted policy interventions to improve educational opportunities, socioeconomic status and healthcare infrastructure to achieve equitable healthcare access for women of childbearing age in Eastern Africa.

2.5 Southern Africa (South Africa)

In Southern Africa, particularly in South Africa, access to reproductive healthcare for women of childbearing age remains an issue of significant concern, even though they had lower maternal mortality compared to other representative regions in Africa that have been reviewed. According to the 2016 DHS Country, the maternal mortality rate was 219 deaths per 100,000 live births, and the maternal mortality ratio was 141 maternal deaths per 100,000 live births [34]. Socioeconomic, cultural and healthcare system factors characterise such indicators. Several studies highlight the multifaceted challenges and varying access points that influence women's reproductive health outcomes.

According to a study conducted in 2015, young women of the 18–24 age group faced significant challenges in accessing and utilising SRH services in Soweto [35]. Although the level of awareness was reported to be good, barriers such as healthcare provider attitudes, poor relations and poor communication with healthcare providers have worsened the problem significantly. Hence, the study recommends youth-friendly services that provide age-appropriate information and support healthy sexual practices to enhance access to SRH services in the area [35].

Regarding improving reproductive outcomes, the prevalence and factors affecting reproductive health outcomes have been reported among South African women [36]. The prevalence rates measured include teenage pregnancy rate (44.4%), HIV prevalence rate (17.1%), sexually transmitted infections rate (40.5%) and female genital schistosomiasis rate (19.7%). The factors contributing to such prevalence levels include early sexual debut, inconsistent contraceptive use and socioeconomic differences. Therefore, the study recommends that addressing the complex relationship between individual behaviours and systemic challenges is relevant to enhancing reproductive healthcare access among such women.

Migration status was another identified factor affecting SRH services among South African women, especially in contraceptive use [37]. Migration status, educational level and knowledge about SRH are critical determinants of contraceptive accessibility and usage [37]. The findings suggest the need for targeted SRH programmes that address the specific needs of migrant populations and promote comprehensive knowledge dissemination [37].

The policy and advocacy landscape surrounding women's reproductive rights in South Africa can influence their access to quality reproductive services [38]. The study showed that the legalisation of abortion contributed to a better way to enhance reproductive utilisation by women of childbearing age in South Africa [38]. However, many oppositions, such as stigma, poor dissemination of information, and an increase in the number of conscientious objectors, to this policy, the Termination of Pregnancy Act, have also impaired the use of safe abortion services, thus leading to an increase in patronage of unsafe abortion services [39]. Therefore, a change in policy can help address the factors that have impeded the progress of improving reproductive healthcare access among women in the nation. Thus, addressing these factors will help improve reproductive healthcare services among women of childbearing age in the country.

Also, community and healthcare providers' opinions on access to reproductive healthcare services have been investigated [40]. The study findings highlight that increasing access to free contraceptive services is hampered by service availability, long waiting times and limited provider training, which are termed structural barriers affecting the access to contraceptive services among women of childbearing age in South Africa [40].

In summary, the current status of reproductive healthcare access in Southern Africa particularly shows a complex interplay of socioeconomic, cultural and systemic factors. Addressing these challenges requires multidimensional approaches, including youth-friendly services, comprehensive SRH education, targeted interventions for migrant populations and policy reforms that safeguard women's reproductive rights and health outcomes. These efforts are crucial for achieving equitable access to reproductive healthcare services and promoting women's overall health and well-being in the region.

3. The significance of improving reproductive healthcare access

Reproductive healthcare is a crucial component of public health, impacting maternal, newborn and child health outcomes globally. Achieving the third Sustainable Development Goal (which aims to ensure the achievement of healthy lives and well-being for all) and universal healthcare coverage (UHC) is intricately linked with improving reproductive healthcare access.

3.1 The need for achieving SDG 3 (ensure the achievement of healthy lives and well-being for all)

3.1.1 Maternal and child health targets

The 3.1 section of SDG 3 sets a goal to reduce the global maternal mortality ratio to less than 70 per 100,000 live births by 2030 [41]. Achieving this global status by many nations of the world, including African countries, lies in enhancing and addressing the barriers affecting women of reproductive age from accessing quality reproductive healthcare services. The World Health Organisation emphasises the need for urgent action, noting that many countries are likely to meet their national targets with significant interventions [41]. Factors contributing to maternal mortality include postpartum haemorrhage, eclampsia, sepsis and unsafe abortion, underscoring the critical need for improved healthcare infrastructure and emergency obstetric care services [42]. Hence, these factors must be addressed to increase access for women of reproductive age to enjoy high-quality healthcare services.

3.1.2 Child health and mortality

Section 3.2 aims to end preventable deaths of newborns and children under 5 years of age, striving for neonatal mortality rates as low as 12 per 1000 live births and under-5 mortality rates as low as 25 per 1000 live births globally by 2030 [41]. This target necessitates comprehensive healthcare strategies to enhance maternal healthcare access, including nutrition services, immunisations, and access to quality maternal and child health services [41]. Therefore, enhancing such access to maternal healthcare services will improve child health and reduce child mortality.

3.1.3 Maternal, newborn, child and adolescent health

Ensuring universal access to sexual and reproductive health services is pivotal in achieving Sustainable Development Goal (SDG) 3.7, which aims to support maternal, newborn, child and adolescent health by promoting comprehensive reproductive healthcare rights and services [41]. This goal recognises that access to such services improves health outcomes and empowers individuals to make informed decisions about their reproductive health, thereby contributing to broader societal well-being [41].

Access to reproductive healthcare services encompasses a spectrum of interventions, including family planning, maternal healthcare and safe abortion services where legal. Family planning, in particular, plays a crucial role in reducing unintended pregnancies, maternal mortality and unsafe abortions [43]. It enables individuals and couples to decide their children's number, timing and spacing, which has long-term implications for maternal and child health outcomes [6].

Despite global commitments, significant disparities in access persist, disproportionately affecting marginalised populations, including women in rural areas, adolescents and those in least developed areas. These disparities are exacerbated by socioeconomic factors, cultural norms and legislative restrictions that limit access to comprehensive reproductive healthcare services [42]. For instance, restrictive laws and policies on abortion hinder access to safe procedures, leading to higher rates of maternal mortality and morbidity in regions with limited healthcare infrastructure [40, 43].

International cooperation and advocacy play crucial roles in advancing reproductive health rights and dismantling barriers to access [41]. By promoting evidence-based policies, supporting health system strengthening and empowering communities to demand and utilise services, stakeholders can accelerate progress towards achieving SDG targets related to maternal, newborn and child health through enhancing access to reproductive healthcare access [41].

The global commitment to SDGs necessitates collaborative efforts across sectors and regions. It has been shown that progress and challenges have been encountered within Gulf Cooperation Council (GCC) states, where initiatives have reduced maternal mortality. However, gaps remain in comprehensive reproductive healthcare access, particularly concerning cultural barriers and disparities in service delivery, especially in the least developed nations in Africa [42].

While substantial effort has been put in place to meet the SDG 3 goal, concerted efforts are needed to bridge gaps in healthcare infrastructure, address socio-cultural barriers and advocate for policy reforms that support comprehensive reproductive healthcare rights and enhance access to reproductive healthcare services for women of reproductive age. By prioritising these efforts, countries, including African nations, can accelerate progress towards achieving SDG 3 and ensuring healthy lives for all.

In summary, expanding access to reproductive healthcare services is a public health imperative and a human rights issue critical for achieving SDG 3 and promoting equitable and sustainable development worldwide. African nations can accomplish these goals by addressing barriers and investing in comprehensive reproductive healthcare to ensure adequate healthcare access is provided for women of childbearing age in their countries.

3.2 The need for achieving universal healthcare coverage (UHC)

Ensuring that every woman has access to reproductive healthcare services is also helpful for accomplishing Universal Healthcare Coverage. The journey towards achieving universal health coverage (UHC) includes improving the availability of essential healthcare services and addressing obstacles that hinder progress in providing reproductive healthcare for women of childbearing age.

3.2.1 Primary healthcare systems

WHO emphasises that sexual and reproductive health (SRH) is integral to health and well-being across the life course and must be embedded within PHC systems for universal access to be achieved [41]. These services not only contribute to reducing maternal mortality and morbidity but also empower individuals to make informed choices about their reproductive health [44].

However, despite global commitments, substantial gaps in SRH service access persist, affecting billions worldwide, particularly women, adolescents and marginalised populations, such as in Africa. Integrating SRH into PHC for UHC requires political commitment, coherent strategies and sufficient resources [41]. Evidence suggests comprehensive SRH services integrated into PHC can improve health outcomes, enhance service delivery efficiency and promote health equity across diverse socio-economic and cultural contexts [44].

The WHO has developed practical tools and resources to support countries in integrating SRH into broader UHC reforms. The Handbook on Integrating SRH within PHC Strategies guides planning, implementing and monitoring of integrated SRH services. It emphasises the importance of aligning national health benefit packages with SRH needs, ensuring service availability and enhancing healthcare provider competencies [41]. This approach enhances service delivery and promotes accountability and inclusivity in healthcare systems.

The Learning by Sharing Portal (LSP) also offers qualitative case studies and best practices from countries worldwide, showcasing innovative approaches to SRH-UHC integration. These examples highlight the role of policy reforms, community engagement and multi-sectoral partnerships in expanding SRH service coverage and improving health outcomes [41].

3.2.2 Challenges and opportunities

Despite progress, several challenges hinder universal access to SRH services. These include policy and legal barriers, inadequate financing, gender inequalities and socio-cultural norms that restrict access to essential SRH interventions like safe abortion services and reproductive cancer care [44]. Addressing these barriers requires sustained advocacy, increased public financing for SRH and strategies to overcome gender-based disparities in service provision.

Evidence indicates that countries with robust PHC systems and inclusive SRH policies achieved better health outcomes and reduced health inequities. For instance, Ireland's approach to strengthening abortion services and Thailand's adoption of health technology assessments for vaccine inclusion demonstrate effective strategies within local contexts [41].

Moving forward, enhancing the priority of SRH within national EPHS and health budgets is crucial for achieving UHC goals. Finding secure and long-lasting funding methods can decrease the need for direct payments, making sexual and reproductive health services more affordable and financially accessible to marginalised communities [44]. Additionally, building alliances among governmental entities, non-governmental organisations and private businesses can utilise resources and knowledge to broaden sexual and reproductive health service availability and enhance service standards.

Additionally, it is crucial to achieve universal health coverage in order to address these disparities and guarantee fair and equal access to vital reproductive health services. This involves enhancing healthcare systems to provide inclusive, affordable and culturally suitable quality services for various populations [41]. Investments in healthcare infrastructure, workforce training and community-based outreach programmes are essential to expanding service delivery and addressing barriers such as geographic isolation and lack of information [6].

In summary, achieving universal access to SRH services through integrated PHC is essential for advancing UHC and fulfilling global health commitments. The WHO's tools and initiatives provide practical frameworks for policymakers, implementers and stakeholders to strengthen SRH service integration, promote health equity and improve health outcomes globally. African countries can adopt the WHO strategies and guidelines to address barriers and invest in comprehensive SRH interventions to facilitate access to reproductive healthcare services among women of childbearing age.

4. Relationship of reproductive healthcare access with healthcare-seeking behaviour

Numerous studies in various geographical areas have highlighted the intricate relationship between the availability of reproductive healthcare and individuals' healthcare-seeking habits. These factors influence a range of socio-cultural, economic and educational factors.

A study carried out among women residing in rural communities in the Haramaya region of East Ethiopia examined the patterns of seeking maternal healthcare [4]. The research results indicated that improving healthcare availability and increasing the utilisation of maternal healthcare services played a crucial role in decreasing maternal illness and death. There is a notable disparity in the utilisation of antenatal care services, hospital deliveries and postnatal care among women. The study reported that educational status, awareness of pregnancy complications and religious beliefs were significant determinants of healthcare-seeking behaviour [4]. Hence, it was suggested that healthcare providers' targeted health education and supportive counselling could enhance maternal healthcare-seeking behaviours [4].

Another study conducted among rural women in Telangana investigated healthcare-seeking behaviour [45]. The study showed poor healthcare-seeking behaviour despite the high awareness among individuals regarding healthcare centres in the study area. Most participants reported that they often visited unqualified healthcare professionals or used home remedies [45]. Therefore, distance to the health facility and improved health behaviour are related to healthcare accessibility. Thus, increasing access to available health centres and access to qualified medical practitioners is essential to enhance positive health-seeking behaviours in rural settings.

Maternal health outcomes in northwest Nigeria, known for having the highest maternal illness and death rates in Africa and globally, have been the subject of research [46]. The research results indicated that various socio-cultural and economic aspects, such as restricted ability to make decisions, deep-seated cultural beliefs, lack of education and limited healthcare access, serve as significant obstacles to using healthcare services [46]. The research suggested taking action to engage husbands, who are often in charge of healthcare decisions within households, and to improve women's access to education in the area.

Envuladu et al. conducted a study on the utilisation of sexual and reproductive health (SRH) services among adolescents in Plateau State, Nigeria [47]. The research discovered that nearly all of the teenagers had not sought out healthcare facilities for sexual and reproductive health (SRH) concerns. Additionally, over half of them expressed unwillingness to seek such help in the future [47]. The main factors contributing to this hesitancy included concerns about privacy and confidentiality, as well as receiving negative attitudes from healthcare providers [47]. The research suggested that enhancing these factors and raising awareness about sexual and reproductive health before initiating sexual activity could potentially boost adolescents' access to sexual and reproductive health services in the area studied [47].

The research emphasises that the utilisation of reproductive healthcare services is closely tied to healthcare-seeking habits, which are greatly affected by educational, socio-cultural and economic aspects. In Ethiopia, a woman's education and understanding of pregnancy complications played a vital role in her decision to seek maternal healthcare services [4]. In Telangana, knowing about the healthcare facilities was crucial but not enough on its own, as it did not address the prevailing dependence on unqualified healthcare providers [45]. The healthcare-seeking behaviours of women in northwest Nigeria are significantly influenced by traditional cultural practices and the dynamics of household decision-making, particularly the influence of husbands [46]. The above studies show that improving women's access to education and including key decision-makers in the household in health initiatives can lead to better utilisation of healthcare services. Adolescents in Plateau State encounter barriers when trying to access sexual and reproductive health services, including challenges related to privacy, confidentiality and healthcare provider attitudes [47]. This emphasises the need for healthcare systems to give more attention to these issues in order to effectively assist adolescents in utilising the services that are available to them.

Therefore, improving access to reproductive healthcare can positively impact women's healthcare-seeking habits when using such services. However, a comprehensive strategy that includes teaching, cultural sensitivity and fundamental modifications in healthcare provision is required. Tailored health education, guidance, involvement of pertinent parties and protecting privacy and confidentiality are crucial methods for improving the accessibility of reproductive healthcare services.

5. Evidence-based recommendations to improve reproductive healthcare access in Africa

Enhancing reproductive healthcare access in Africa necessitates a comprehensive approach, as underscored by various studies. These studies identify effective interventions, challenges and strategies for scaling up access to reproductive healthcare services.

5.1 Youth-friendly health services/adolescent health services in Nigeria

Youth-Friendly Health Services (YFHS) represents a cost-effective approach/intervention to addressing the sexual and reproductive health needs of young individuals in sub-Saharan Africa (SSA) [48]. Their review identifies significant implementation strategies: stakeholder training, infrastructure modification and consumer engagement. The study showed that YFHS interventions were effective; however, optimisation and sustainability of these interventions in resource-limited settings, such as Africa [48], are required. The implementation of YFHS can be achieved by channelling the strategies to specific contexts and regularly evaluating their effectiveness and sustainability. In addition, another study has investigated four Nigerian states integrating adolescent and youth-friendly health services (AYFHS) within a systems-based approach [49]. The study showed that implementing a streamlined quality assurance (QA) tool and follow-up quality improvement (QI) activities achieved significant improvements in contraceptive services for adolescents and youth. Training providers and using quality assurance/quality improvement tools within supportive supervision systems can effectively enhance the quality and uptake of AYFHS [49].

5.2 Maternal health interventions

A systematic review study that offers a realist synthesis of maternal health interventions in low- and middle-income countries shows helpful interventions that can help enhance maternal health outcomes [50]. The study underscores the significance of healthcare system infrastructure in the success of these interventions. Effective interventions often involve increasing knowledge and awareness among individuals and healthcare providers regarding maternal health [50]. The study also emphasises the importance of engaging communities and families to address social and cultural norms that influence healthcare-seeking behaviours [50].

5.3 Reforming primary health care

A review of interventions aimed at improving primary healthcare (PHC) for maternal, newborn and child health (MNCH) in SSA has been conducted [51]. Effective strategies include financial incentives, task-shifting, community-directed engagements and mobile health. The review suggests that to improve access to and quality of PHC services, these interventions must be scaled up and sustained through appropriate policies and programmes [51]. The findings provide valuable insights into reforming PHC systems to enhance regional MNCH outcomes. Also, adopting the practical tool offered by the WHO can be beneficial. The Handbook on Integrating SRH within PHC Strategies guides planning, implementing, and monitoring of integrated SRH services. It emphasises the importance of aligning national health benefit packages with SRH needs, ensuring service availability and enhancing healthcare provider competencies [41].

5.4 Institutionalising health technology assessment

The role of health technology assessment (HTA) in designing health benefit packages for sexual and reproductive health and rights (SRHR) has been identified as an effective intervention to improving reproductive healthcare access [52]. The study highlights the need for stakeholder participation and standardised assessment processes to ensure fair and effective SRHR interventions. Institutionalising HTA and establishing clear decision-making criteria can help integrate diverse social values and improve SRHR outcomes [52].

5.5 Promoting task sharing for family planning

Implementing task sharing for family planning in five sub-Saharan African countries was reviewed by Ouedraogo et al. [53]. The study found that involving community health workers, midwives and nurses in delivering contraceptive services significantly increased the contraceptive uptake rate. Despite the success, poor provider retention and inadequate documentation persist [53]. Task-sharing is a promising strategy to enhance family planning services, but it requires robust policy frameworks and effective data systems for sustainability.

Therefore, to enhance reproductive healthcare access in Africa, evidence-based strategies must address the unique needs and challenges of the region. Thus, considering the identified evidence-based interventions (Youth-Friendly Health Services/ Adolescent Health Services in Nigeria, maternal health interventions, reforming primary healthcare, institutionalising health technology assessment, promoting task-sharing for family planning) will help in enhancing reproductive healthcare access, reducing maternal mortality and improving the achievement of SDG 3 and UHC global goals in African nations.

6. Conclusion

This chapter has discussed comprehensively the theme of enhancing reproductive healthcare access for women of childbearing age in Africa. It highlighted the current status of reproductive healthcare access in Africa by using maternal mortality metrics and evidence from existing studies that have highlighted the factors influencing reproductive healthcare access among women of childbearing age. It discussed the importance of reproductive healthcare access in achieving SDG 3 and UHC. In addition, it showed that a positive relationship exists between reproductive health access and health-seeking behaviours using evidence from published studies. It finally identified five recommendations that will help enhance access to reproductive healthcare access among women of reproductive age, which African nations can adopt based on the unique challenges of the region.

Acknowledgements

I want to extend my sincere appreciation to my former master's supervisor and current co-author, Professor Charles Tobin-West, for his guidance, support, corrections, feedback, and constructive criticism throughout the development of this chapter despite his tight schedule. I would also like to express my heartfelt gratitude to my parents (Mr. and Mrs. David Ngweeh), Siblings (Jonathan, Bethel, & Kingsley) and friends (Samson, Rejoice, Salvation, Oyiza, and Frank) for their unwavering support and encouragement throughout this journey.

Conflict of interest

The authors declare no conflict of interest.

Thanks

Thank you, IntechOpen, for deeming us worthy of contributing to this global project. I look forward to future opportunities for collaboration.

Author details

Japheth David* and Charles Tobin-West
Department of Preventive and Social Medicine, University of Port Harcourt, Port Harcourt, Nigeria

*Address all correspondence to: davidjapheth6@gmail.com; japheth_david@uniport.edu.ng

References

[1] WHO. Maternal mortality rate: The urgency of a systemic and multisectoral approach in mitigating maternal deaths in Africa. 2023. Available from: https://files.aho.afro.who.int/afahobckpcontainer/production/files/iAHO_Maternal_Mortality_Regional_Factsheet.pdf [Accessed: July 4, 2024]

[2] Dahab R, Sakellariou D. Barriers to accessing maternal care in low income countries in Africa: A systematic review. International Journal of Environmental Research and Public Health. 2020;**17**:4292. DOI: 10.3390/ijerph17124292

[3] Ogundele OJ, Pavlova M, Groot W. Inequalities in reproductive health care use in five West-African countries: A decomposition analysis of the wealth-based gaps. International Journal of Equity in Health. 2020;**19**:44

[4] Kifle D, Azale T, Gelaw YA, Melsew YA. Maternal health care service seeking behaviours and associated factors among women in rural Haramaya district, Eastern Ethiopia: A triangulated community-based cross-sectional study. Reproductive Health. 2017;**14**:1-11. DOI: 10.1186/s12978-016-0270-5

[5] WHO. Maternal mortality. 2024b. Available from: https://www.who.int/news-room/fact-sheets/detail/maternal-mortality/?gad_source=1&gclid=CjwKCAjw7s20BhBFEiwABVIMrQq58jcxIVnP3X2nRHgRMtdOUCYO22MSnSw1BIW1rBrkk NWhqPhrZxoCL7QQAvD_BwE [Accessed: July 4, 2024]

[6] UNICEF. Maternal mortality. 2023. Available from: https://data.unicef.org/topic/maternal-health/maternal-mortality/ [Accessed: July 4, 2024]

[7] Samuel O, Zewotir T, North D. Decomposing the urban-rural inequalities in the utilisation of maternal health care services: Evidence from 27 selected countries in sub-Saharan Africa. Reproductive Health. 2021;**18**:216

[8] Statista. African countries with the largest population in 2023. 2023. Available from: https://www.statista.com/statistics/1121246/population-in-africa-by-country/ [Accessed: July 4, 2024]

[9] National Geographic Society. Africa: Human geography. 2023. Available from: https://education.nationalgeographic.org/resource/africa-human-geography/ [Accessed: July 4, 2024]

[10] Ministry of Health and Population (Egypt), El-Zanaty and Associates, and ICF International. Egypt Demographic and Health Survey 2014. Cairo, Egypt: Ministry of Health and Population and ICF International; 2015

[11] Abdel-Tawab N, Rabie T, Boehmova Z, Hawkins L, Saher S, El-Shitany A. Do public health services in Egypt help young married women exercise their reproductive rights? International Journal of Gynecology and Obstetrics. 2015;**130**:E52-E55. DOI: 10.1016/j.ijgo.2015.03.012

[12] Metwally AM, Saleh RM, El-Etreby LA, Salama SI, Aboulghate A, Amer HA, et al. Enhancing the value of women's reproductive rights through community-based interventions in upper Egypt governorates: A randomised interventional study. International Journal for Equity in Health. 2019;**18**:1. DOI: 10.1186/s12939-019-1042-y

[13] Samari G. Education and fertility in Egypt: Mediation by women's empowerment. SSM—Population Health. 2019;**9**:1-9. DOI: 10.1016/j.ssmph.2019.100488

[14] Aly RAM. Empowerment as a mediator between education and reproductive health care in Egypt: The impact of poverty and residence. Open Journal of Social Sciences. 2021;**09**:58-76. DOI: 10.4236/jss.2021.93005

[15] Elsayed R, Zembe-Mkabile W. Women's access to sexual and reproductive health services and information in Ismailia, Egypt. BMC Women's Health. 2024;**24**:1-11. DOI: 10.1186/s12905-024-02986-4

[16] National Population Commission (Nigeria) and ICF International. Nigeria Demographic and Health Survey 2018. Abuja, Nigeria: National Population Commission and ICF International; 2019

[17] Ayanleye OA. Women and reproductive health rights in Nigeria. OIDA International Journal of Sustainable Development. 2013;**6**:127-140

[18] Agbor IM. Access to reproductive health-care services and its impact on the health of women in Guma local government area, Benue state, Nigeria. Journal of Social and Political Sciences. 2020;**3**:419-438. DOI: 10.31014/aior.1991.03.02.180

[19] Bolarinwa OA, Fortune E, Aboagye RG, Seidu AA, Olagunju OS, Nwagbara UI, et al. Health facility delivery among women of reproductive age in Nigeria: Does age at first birth matter? PLoS One. 2021;**16**:11. DOI: 10.1371/journal.pone.0259250

[20] Public Services International. Linking sexual and reproductive health with gender-transformative quality public services the global union federation of workers in public services. 2023. Available from: https://publicservices.international/resources/publications/linking-sexual-and-reproductive-health-with-gender-transformative-quality-public-services?id=14303&lang=en [Accessed: July 4, 2024]

[21] Sule ST, Dieng B, Danmadami AM. Reproductive health issues of concern among Nigerians: An online survey. International Journal of Community Medicine and Public Health. 2023;**1**:104-110. DOI: 10.18203/2394-6040.ijcmph20234114

[22] Omokwe MM. Maternal healthcare service utilisation in Abia South Senatorial district, Nigeria: Urban-rural differences of maternal healthcare service utilisation in Abia South Senatorial district, Abia state, Nigeria. The Nigerian Health Journal. 2024;**24**:1047-1057. DOI: 10.60787/tnhj.v24i1.763

[23] Ministère du Plan et Suivi de la Mise en Œuvre de la Révolution de la Modernité (Democratic Republic of Congo), Ministère de la Santé Publique, and ICF International. Enquête Démographique et de Santé en République Démocratique du Congo 2013-14. Kinshasa, Democratic Republic of Congo: Ministère du Plan et Suivi de la Mise en Œuvre de la Révolution de la Modernité and ICF International; 2014

[24] Kwete D, Binanga A, Mukaba T, Nemuandjare T, Mbadu MF, Kyungu MT, et al. Family planning in the Democratic Republic of the Congo: Encouraging momentum, formidable challenges. Global Health: Science and Practice. 2018;**6**:40-54. DOI: 10.9745/GHSP-D-17-00346

[25] Butler MG, Walker M, Pablo LA, Bartels SA. Relationship between

women's decision-making power over their own health care and use of modern contraception in the Democratic Republic of the Congo: A cross-sectional secondary data analysis. BMC Women's Health. 2021;**21**:1-13. DOI: 10.1186/s12905-021-01450-x

[26] Glover AL, Mulunda JC, Akilimali P, Kayembe D, Bertrand JT. Expanding access to safe abortion in DRC: Charting the path from decriminalisation to accessible care. Sexual and Reproductive Health Matters. 2023;**31**:1-12. DOI: 10.1080/26410397.2023.2273893

[27] Ibrahimi S, Youssouf B, Potts C, Dumouza A, Duff R, Malaba LS, et al. United States government-supported family planning and reproductive health outreach in the Democratic Republic of the Congo: Lessons learned and recommendations. Open Access Journal of Contraception. 2024;**15**:13-21. DOI: 10.2147/oajc.s446263

[28] Central Statistical Agency (Ethiopia) and ICF International. Ethiopia Demographic and Health Survey 2016. Addis Ababa, Ethiopia: Central Statistical Agency and ICF International; 2017

[29] Fetene SM, Haile TG. Three-fourths of women of reproductive age in emerging regions of Ethiopia are facing problems in accessing health care. Scientific Reports. 2023;**13**:1-10. DOI: 10.1038/s41598-023-36223-z

[30] Darebo TD, Birhanu Z, Alemayehu M, Balcha B, Worku A, Assele DD, et al. Utilisation of sexual and reproductive health services among construction worker women in southern Ethiopia. BMC Women's Health. 2024;**24**:1-10. DOI: 10.1186/s12905-024-03042-x

[31] Handebo S, Demie TG, Woldeamanuel BT, Biratu TD, Gessese GT. Enrollment of reproductive age women in community-based health insurance: An evidence from 2019 mini Ethiopian demographic and health survey. Frontiers in Public Health. 2023;**11**:1-9. DOI: 10.3389/fpubh.2023.1067773

[32] Tamirat KS, Tessema ZT, Kebede FB. Factors associated with the perceived barriers of health care access among reproductive-age women in Ethiopia: A secondary data analysis of 2016 Ethiopian demographic and health survey. BMC Health Services Research. 2020;**20**:1-8

[33] Zegeye B, Adjei NK, Ahinkorah BO, Ameyaw EK, Budu E, Seidu AA, et al. Barriers and facilitators to accessing health care services among married women in Ethiopia: A multi-level analysis of the Ethiopia demographic and health survey. International Journal of Translational Medical Research and Public Health. 2021;**5**:183-196. DOI: 10.21106/ijtmrph.380

[34] Statistics South Africa and National Department of Health (South Africa). South Africa Demographic and Health Survey, 2016. Pretoria, South Africa: Statistics South Africa and National Department of Health; 2017

[35] Lince-Deroche N, Hargey A, Holt K, Shochet T. Accessing sexual and reproductive health information and services: A mixed methods study of young women's needs and experiences in Soweto, South Africa. African Journal of Reproductive Health. 2015;**19**:73

[36] Galappaththi-Arachchige HN, Zulu SG, Kleppa E, Lillebo K, Qvigstad E, Ndhlovu P, et al. Reproductive health problems in rural South African young women: Risk behaviour and risk factors. Reproductive Health. 2018;**15**:1-10. DOI: 10.1186/s12978-018-0581-9

[37] Chawhanda C, Levin J, Ibisomi L. Factors associated with sexual and reproductive health service utilisation in high migration communities in six Southern African countries. BMC Public Health. 2022;**22**:1-15. DOI: 10.1186/s12889-022-13308-4

[38] Mbali M, Mthembu S. The politics of women's health in South Africa. Agenda. 2012;**26**:4-14. DOI: 10.1080/10130950.2012.714674

[39] Favier M, Greenberg JMS, Stevens M. Safe abortion in South Africa: "We have wonderful laws but we don't have people to implement those laws". International Journal of Gynecology and Obstetrics. 2018;**143**:38-44. DOI: 10.1002/ijgo.12676

[40] Kriel Y, Milford C, Cordero JP, Suleman F, Steyn PS, Smit JA. Access to public sector family planning services and modern contraceptive methods in South Africa: A qualitative evaluation from community and health care provider perspectives. PLoS One. 2023;**18**:1-20. DOI: 10.1371/journal.pone.0282996

[41] WHO. Accelerating progress towards reducing maternal, newborn and child mortality in order to achieve sustainable development goal targets 3.1 and 3.2.2024. Available from: https://www.who.int/publications/m/item/wha-agenda-item-11.7—accelerate-progress-towards-reducing-maternal--newborn-and-child-mortality-in-order-to-achieve-sdg-targets-3.1-and-3.2 [Accessed: July 4, 2024]

[42] Daher-Nashif S, Bawadi H. Women's health and well-being in the United Nations sustainable development goals: A narrative review of achievements and gaps in the Gulf states. International Journal of Environmental Research and Public Health. 2020;**17**:1-8. DOI: 10.3390/ijerph17031059

[43] Espey E, Dennis A, Landy U. The importance of access to comprehensive reproductive health care, including abortion: A statement from women's health professional organisations. American Journal of Obstetrics and Gynecology. 2019;**220**:67-70. DOI: 10.1016/j.ajog.2018.09.008

[44] Ravindran TKS, Govender V. Sexual and reproductive health services in universal health coverage: A review of recent evidence from low- and middle-income countries. Sexual and Reproductive Health Matters. 2020;**28**:1-22. DOI: 10.1080/26410397.2020.1779632

[45] PmC R, Rineetha T, Sreeharshika D, Jothula K. Health care seeking behaviour among rural women in Telangana: A cross-sectional study. Journal of Family Medicine and Primary Care. 2020;**9**:4778. DOI: 10.4103/jfmpc.jfmpc_489_20

[46] Kubra-Hassan H, Adamu-Basirka I. Healthcare seeking behavior and utilization of maternal healthcare services among women of reproductive age in Northwest, Nigeria. Gusau International Journal of Management and Social Sciences. 2021;**4**:1-17

[47] Envuladu EA, Massar K, de Wit J. Adolescents sexual and reproductive healthcare-seeking behaviour and service utilisation in plateau state, Nigeria. Healthcare (Switzerland). 2022;**10**:1-10. DOI: 10.3390/healthcare10020301

[48] Obiezu-Umeh C, Nwaozuru U, Mason S, Gbaja-Biamila T, Oladele D, Ezechi O, et al. Implementation strategies to enhance youth-friendly sexual and reproductive health services in sub-Saharan Africa: A systematic review. Frontiers in Reproductive Health. Frontiers Media S.A. 2021;**3**:1-13. DOI: 10.3389/frph.2021.684081

[49] Akila D, Oluwasegun A, Bose K, Omotoso O, Adefila A, Mwaikambo L. Improving the quality of adolescent and youth-friendly health services through integrated supportive supervision in four Nigerian states key findings. Global Health, Science and Practice. 2024;**12**:e2200169. DOI: 10.9745/GHSP-D-22-00169

[50] Abraham JM, Melendez-Torres GJ. A realist review of interventions targeting maternal health in low- and middle-income countries. Women's Health. 2023;**19**:1-12. DOI: 10.1177/17455057231205687

[51] Okonofua FE, Ntoimo LFC, Adejumo OA, Imongan W, Ogu RN, Anjorin SO. Assessment of interventions in primary health care for improved maternal, newborn and child health in sub-Saharan Africa: A systematic review. SAGE Open. 2022;**12**:1-19. DOI: 10.1177/21582440221134222

[52] Simangolwa WM, Mbonigaba J, Govender K. Health technology assessment for sexual reproductive health and rights benefits package design in sub-Saharan Africa: A scoping review of evidence-informed deliberative processes. PLoS One. 2024;**19**:e0306042. DOI: 10.1371/journal.pone.0306042

[53] Ouedraogo L, Habonimana D, Nkurunziza T, Chilanga A, Hayfa E, Fatim T, et al. Towards achieving the family planning targets in the African region: A rapid review of task sharing policies. Reproductive Health. 2021;**18**:1-12. DOI: 10.1186/s12978-020-01038-y

Chapter 7

Collaborative Care for Health Equity: Integrated Care for Underserved Populations

Theresa Abah and Ifeyinwa Onwelumadu

Abstract

Collaborative care for health equity aims to integrate primary and hospital care to serve clients. Drawing insights from various practices and research behind the continued struggle of underserved communities, and the root causes of health inequities and institutional failures, the chapter unveils how collaborative care integrates primary and hospital care to serve people better. The approaches highlighted show that meaningful improvements in health outcomes, require addressing both medical and social determinants of health particularly for underserved communities. Some of the causative conditions of inequity, such as, unaddressed social determinants of health, exacerbated by issues of low income, race/ethnicity and other environmental factors increase the disproportionate experiences of patients. It provides a way forward to achieve health equity by emphasizing, income, race, education and professional ethics as part of the decision-making processes needed for equitable healthcare. Addressing inequities in healthcare access among individuals at a higher risk for mortality and morbidity from all forms of systemic issues will reduce illnesses and improve access to healthcare especially issues bedeviling the health systems globally. Overall, understanding these issues will help to develop practical steps to improve healthcare access and discourage the focus on episodic reaction to health care.

Keywords: health inequities, underserved populations, hospital access, healthcare disparities, cultural competency, collaborative care models, integrated healthcare

1. Introduction

Collaborative care for health equity aims to integrate primary and hospital care to serve population subgroups effectively, with special focus on underserved populations. This approach recognizes that meaningful improvements in health outcomes, particularly for marginalized communities, require addressing both medical and social determinants of health. While a number of studies suggest a need for multidisciplinary team of professionals to achieve collaborative care using innovative approaches, policy reform and effective coordination of resources, others suggest that successful implementation of collaborative care models depends on political will and addressing the multi-level factors that enhance healthcare access.

The World Health Organization report in 2021 estimates that about 4.5 billion people do not receive enough health care service that they need globally, while in the United States, about 1 in 10 people are without health insurance. These issues and other unaddressed social determinants of health in healthcare delivery hinders access to care for underserved populations. Enhanced healthcare access is shown to be associated with the effective utilization of tools that promote collaboration opportunities and appropriate interventions that among stakeholders [1–4]. Achieving health equity for all- where all individuals therefore, would require that everyone have the opportunity to attain their full health potential, and this remains a critical challenge in the healthcare landscape. Integrated care models which promote care coordination and collaboration among primary and hospital systems present an opportunity to address this disproportionate healthcare landscape especially among underserved people.

Integrated care systems significantly contribute to improving care access, availability, affordability, and acceptability of healthcare services for all population subgroups [5, 6]. This chapter will analyze how health systems improve healthcare access by shedding light on some steps to implement collaborative care teams at the community level, it also provides measures for evaluating success and service delivery. Integrated primary, specialty and hospital-based care models provide a more comprehensive, patient-centered approach to addressing the multifaceted health needs of underserved populations [7, 8]. While some key metrics for measuring the impact of collaborative care are listed in this chapter, it is necessary to highlight some benefits in the examples in **Table 1**, such as, ability to implement cost-effective care, promote health equity, reduce inequalities and promote healthcare access [11, 14, 16, 17]. In sum, the chapter provides steps to achieve collaborative care to deliver optimal health and provide ways to address access to care among population subgroups.

2. Learning objectives

1. After reviewing this chapter, the reader should be able to complete the following:

2. Evaluate the impact of integrated care models on health outcomes for underserved populations.

3. Analyze strategies to increase accessibility to preventive health services in underserved communities.

4. Assess the effectiveness of initiatives aimed at enhancing patient experience and reducing healthcare costs in underserved areas.

5. Design community-based interventions to promote health equity for underserved groups.

6. Critique the coordination mechanisms between primary and hospital care for their effectiveness in serving underserved populations.

7. Synthesize interprofessional collaborative practices to support comprehensive care in underserved communities and develop data-driven approaches to identify and address healthcare access gaps.

Integrated framework/ author	Area of integration	Strategy	Lessons learned	Challenges
Integrated Collaborative Care Team (ICCT) Joanna L. Henderson et al. [9].	Better youth Mental Health Access (MHA) outcomes	Integration of community health workers (CHWs) into healthcare teams	Better MHA are anticipated when a quick, stepped-care strategy tailored to need is implemented in a setting that is welcoming to young people.	service delivery gap for youths with MHA challenges in Ontario's current health system structure
The Quadruple Aim Valaitis et al. [10].	Improving patient experience, reducing cost, advancing population health and improving the provider experience in Canada	Ten case studies were conducted in three provinces (Nova Scotia, Ontario, and British Columbia) to elucidate experiences of primary care and public health collaboration in different settings, contexts,	Cases achieved outcomes addressing the Q-Aims such as improving access to services, addressing population health through outreach to at-risk populations, reducing costs through efficiencies, and improving provider	Common precipitators were having a shared vision and/or community concern. Barriers and enablers differed among cases. Perceived barriers included ineffective communication processes,
Community-based Cosupervisory Model Gunderson JM et al. [11].	Community health workers, extension of care coordination	Description of collaborative development of community-based CHW program to address the social determinants of health that affect patients	The cosupervisory, generalist CHW model provides an innovative template for cocreation of patient-centered infrastructure and resourcing within an evolving and replicable holistic care continuum	Building sustainable interdisciplinary relationships
Conceptual Integrated Care Model (CICM) M. H. Chin et al. [7].	Government and private policies, health equity	Developed a conceptual model that highlights how government and private policies influence health equity by impacting the healthcare system (access to care, structure and quality of care, payment of care), and	To authentically commit to achieving health equity, nations should: (1) Explicitly design quality of care and payment policies to achieve equity, holding the healthcare system accountable through public	Ability to conduct self-evaluation to address implicit bias by adopters of the policy
Population Health Equity Framework Trinh-Shevrin et al. [12]	Health Promotion and Disease Prevention	We describe the concepts and parallel approaches that underpin an integrative population health equity framework and present the experience of NYU Center for the Study of Asian American Health	Applying an integrative framework has deepened our community engagement efforts, our understanding of the multi-level contextual factors that influence health, and our capacity to advance	Understanding the multi-factoral context that promote health equity

Integrated framework/ author	Area of integration	Strategy	Lessons learned	Challenges
Community of solution Ferrer et al. [13]	Advanced primary care, health among people living in poverty	The community of solution comprises a county health system, a family medicine residency program, a metropolitan public health department, and local nonprofit organizations and businesses.	Population-based outcome metrics include reductions in hospitalizations, emergency department and urgent care visits, and the associated charges. Promotors also assess patients'	The major challenge noted is the need for training and retraining of health professionals to implement the strategy as required, leading to a high cost of healthcare in the long run
Quality improvement collaboratives (QICs) based on the Chronic Care Model (CCM) Grossman et al. [14].	Community health centers (CHCs)	Describe initiatives undertaken by community health centers (CHCs) participating in QICs (the Health Disparities Collaboratives) for asthma, cardiovascular disease, or diabetes, and to determine whether	Participating CHCs undertook an average of 44 QI activities per center (range, 8–84). These interventions were distributed broadly throughout the elements of the CCM, with particular emphasis on patient	It remains unclear how specific activities pursued under the guidance of the CCM and QICs contribute to quality improvement.
World Health Organization Integrated Care for Older People with Frailty (ICOPE) WHO ICOPE Araujo De Carvalho et al. [15].	Integrate health and social service care to support older people health and wellbeing	Health systems and services organized and coordinated to meet the needs and preferences and goals of older adults	Integrating health and social services entails providing comprehensive assessment and case management considered as an effective approach that targets management of multiple morbidity	Concept of integrated care interventions focus mostly on hospitalization, mortality, physical functioning rather than on all aspects of wellbeing

Table 1.
List of integrated frameworks in practice.

3. Enhancing healthcare access

According to the World Health Organization report on health equity, "*Knowledge, monitoring and analysis are the backbone of actions needed to achieve equity*" [5]. Collaborative care systems have the potential to significantly improve healthcare access for underserved populations [7, 18, 19]. These systems integrate primary and hospital care, bridging traditional service delivery silos and coordinating medical and non-medical services to address the complex needs of high-risk, high-cost individuals [6]. Although there are challenges to achieving a seamless coordination between health systems in areas of workforce training, communication among providers, infrastructural gaps, policy issues, etc. Analyzing the impact of collaborative care in research, it can be deduced that this leads to improved patient outcomes, reduced wait times, and better appointment availability. Integrated care models prioritize community-level collaboration and person-centered care, which is particularly effective in promoting long-term health equity [16, 20]. Key metrics for measuring the impact of these models include reduced hospital readmissions, increased preventive care utilization, improved patient satisfaction and quality of life [16, 21]. From a cost-effectiveness perspective, the upfront implementation burden of collaborative care programs is often offset by long-term healthcare savings through reduced emergency department visits, inpatient hospitalizations, and overall healthcare utilization [1, 16, 22]. These studies provide suggestions on how to sustain this practice, one common strategy is to integrate social (SDOH) determinants of health as a major factor for adopting collaborative care in practice. By considering people's SDOH, policy makers factor patients from underserved communities in resource allocation and distribution which in turn yields significant returns on investment and support a sustainable, equitable healthcare system. In addition, integrating SDOH in care delivery not only enhance access but also factors people's unique qualities, thus, addressing the imbalances in healthcare. This approach focuses on distributing resources based on individual/community needs to achieve fair outcomes.

3.1 Integrated/collaborative care: Addressing health outcomes and equity

The integration of clinical care and public health has become increasingly recognized as a crucial strategy to address local health needs and improve overall health outcomes. Discussions on collaborative care between clinical practice and public health helps to highlight the importance of cross-sectoral collaboration, emphasizing the need for optimal healthcare delivery, and for health systems to tackle specific health challenges [13, 15]. Studies that explored how public health decisions could be incorporated into clinical practice suggest there should be collaboration at all levels of implementation (that is, at institutional, organizational, community and individual levels) to ensure access, fairness, safety and quality of care. Some successful frameworks reviewed include, Conceptual Integrated Care Model (CICM), Community-based Co-Supervisory Model (CBCM), the "Quadruple Aims", "Integrated Collaborative Care Team (ICCT)", "Community of Solutions, Quality Improvement Collaboratives (QICs)" and "WHO Integrated Care for older People with frailty (ICOPE)", [4, 11, 13, 16, 18, 22–24]. These frameworks examine improvement in patient experience and system improvement, suggesting that, integrating care helps to reduce costs, advance population health, improve quality of care, safety, fairness as well as enhance provider experience. Another example of integrated clinical care with community-focused intervention highlight the benefits of providing adequate resources as a key strategy to providing equitable care. Ferrer and colleagues describe a community-based approach in care delivery aimed at improving health outcomes for low-income populations. This model consists of a team of stakeholders including family medicine program, county health system, public health department and local non-profit businesses and organizations. The strategy employed addressed social determinants of health (SDOH) such as (socioeconomic status, education, housing, and access to nutritious food), in the community of solution practice to improve health outcomes. The integration of these SDOH into healthcare delivery is considered essential to effectively serving underserved populations and improve health outcomes [11, 23]. Although there are recorded challenges in the cost of investing in integrated care among hospital and primary care providers, such as setback in underinvestment, which is mostly associated to the short-term benefits these providers stand to make in establishing their business, rather than the long-term community health benefits. Overall, there is much more to be gained from integrated and collaborative partnership approach when the focus is placed on, understanding people's SDOH as a crucial factor to achieve health equity.

Gunderson and colleagues in their study underscore the important role of community health workers as a crucial addition in extending primary care access using a community-based models. The strategy addressed social determinants of health of communities as a vehicle to promote health equity [4, 23]. The growing momentum for multisector collaboration to address social determinants of health is reflected in various initiatives, as highlighted above. These efforts acknowledge that creating healthier environments requires action beyond the traditional boundaries of public health and healthcare, necessitating the collective efforts of various sectors to improve the conditions for achieving healthcare access and well-being. In the same context, other authors like Castillo and colleagues reviewed effective community interventions for promoting mental health and social equity, emphasizing the importance of multi-sector partnerships and community involvement in achieving these goals [17]. The authors suggest that, improving access to mental health care requires integrating mental health services into community organizations including schools, primary care clinics, prisons, etc., particularly for underserved populations whose access to specialized mental health services may be impeded. As a whole, overall health outcome result from the early detection and treatment of mental health disorders made possible by this integration. This strategy helped to address stigma in mental care service, holistic care, patient satisfaction, rapid access to services as a result promoting social justice among underserved groups. Similarly, there's been a focus on preventing chronic diseases through the integration of public health into healthcare systems. Addressing the social determinants of health and the need for a community-oriented, collaborative approach [14]. The integration of clinical care and public health, facilitated by factors such as flexible financing, shared leadership, shared data, and a strong shared vision, holds the potential to bridge traditional service delivery silos and deliver person-centered, holistic care that addresses the complex needs of high-risk, high-cost individuals [20, 25].

Achieving health equity, where all individuals have the opportunity to attain their full health potential, remains a critical challenge in the healthcare landscape. Integrated care models, aim to promote the coordination and collaboration of primary and hospital-based care, and this approach presents a promising approach to reducing health disparities among underserved populations [16, 17, 26]. Lack of access to quality healthcare is a key driver of health inequities, thus integrating primary, specialty, and hospital-based care models hold the potential to providing a more comprehensive, patient-centered approach to care that addresses the multifaceted health needs of underserved populations [7, 27]. The studies in **Table 1** adopt collaborative approaches which highlight the benefits of community involvement and the inclusion of social determinants of health as part of health policy to improving population health outcomes and promote health equity.

4. Frameworks for bridging the equity gap

Conceptual frameworks provide detailed outline of strategies adopted to improve population health outcomes through the lens of collaborative effort among different stakeholders (See **Table 1**). The key points summarized from the given contexts are as follows: In order to have a long-lasting effect on community health, the authors propose a widely applicable strategy for health systems to promote population health in the fields of practice, education, and research. - To address health disparities and improve health outcomes, the strategy involves a wide range of stakeholders, including a county health system, a family medicine residency program, the public health department, and nearby nonprofit organizations and businesses. The Table describe evidence-based frameworks on collaborative care to advance equity in population health. The authors describe methods for increasing access to services and the partnerships to achieve the desired outcomes. For example, the case study from the NYU Center for the Study of Asian American Health (CSAAH) demonstrate how this framework was instrumental to improving health equity among Asian American communities with – "Promotors" (also known as community health workers), including the vital role they played in optimizing community health using this framework. The Promotors carry out neighborhood-specific, and individual-based community-based interventions, concentrating on utilizing family and community resources to assist patients in reaching their health goals. The authors emphasize the importance of population-based outcome measures, such as reductions in hospitalizations and ER visits [18].

These conceptual frameworks also emphasize the need to implement integrated care models that considers peoples' social determinants of health (SDOH) to advance health equity and reduce disparities as well as improve population health outcomes [16]. Integrated care approaches address multi-level contextual factors that underpins health inequities, by coordinating clinical interventions across various care settings to help mitigate the systemic barriers that contribute to health disparities. According to the WHO report on integrated care, frameworks that considers people's functional abilities, disability and other SDOH factors are essential to understanding the complex interplay between health disparities, health equity, social justice, and their influence on access to care [24]. Further highlighting the unique challenges faced by individuals from underserved jurisdictions, such as, the elderly and people from diverse ethnic backgrounds. Collaborative care can specifically address these needs by tailoring interventions to improve access, enhance communication, and provide comprehensive support services. For instance, these models incorporate assistive technologies to provide specialized training for healthcare providers, and ensure physical accessibility of healthcare facilities [10, 24, 28, 29]. By focusing on these multi-faceted strategies, collaborative care can significantly improve healthcare experiences and outcomes for people from all backgrounds. Moreover, collaborative care models can improve the functional capacity and overall well-being of populations by providing a holistic view of a more comprehensive view of the potential benefits and strategies for successful implementation of care that is equitable. Thus, addressing not just medical care needs, but also functional and social needs and enhance the quality of life.

5. Ethical and professional considerations

The pursuit of health equity through integrated care models needs careful consideration of ethical and professional responsibilities. Cultural competency is vital to promote respect and effectively serve diverse cultural backgrounds. The ability of healthcare professionals to provide quality care while honoring and recognizing cultural differences is not only important, but entails being conscious of one's own prejudices, to comprehend how a patient's culture shapes their perceptions of their health, realizing the dynamics of power and privilege, and offering care that is appropriate for the patient's culture. Including cultural competency as part of the training needs for healthcare providers ensures respect and effectively addressing the diverse cultural backgrounds of patients. For example, India in a study that examines a strategy for reducing ethnic and racial disparity in care in the U.S. emphasized that cultural competency can help minorities receive higher-quality care, which will reduce health disparities by encouraging effective communication and patient participation in decision-making [19]. Also, Moore and colleagues argue that all individuals will participate more in clinical trials if appropriately trained nurses and nurse practitioners from a variety of backgrounds are included. Promoting participation regardless of socioeconomic or demographic characteristics and inform patients about trials and ways to lower personal barriers [20]. In sum, clinicians and healthcare organizations who ensure that integrated care initiatives do not inadvertently exacerbate existing biases or introduce new forms of discrimination and respect different cultural norms and practices, are more likely to provide culturally sensitive care that is appropriate. Collection of patient information should be based on their consent and obtained in a way that is clear and comprehensible to patients, for example, respecting their autonomy and right to make informed decisions about their care. Additionally, maintaining patient confidentiality is central especially in communities where trust in the healthcare system may be fragile. Protecting patient information and ensuring privacy, help to build and maintain trust between healthcare providers and patients [20]. Ongoing evaluation and adjustment of these models, with input from diverse stakeholders, are crucial to upholding the principles of justice, beneficence, and non-maleficence.

5.1 Professional roles and responsibilities

Exploring the professional roles and responsibilities of care providers within a collaborative care framework is essential for ensuring equitable and high-quality care for all. Healthcare providers must work effectively in interdisciplinary teams, sharing responsibility for patient outcomes and maintaining clear communication with patients and their families. This involves understanding and respecting the scope of practice of different team members and fostering a cooperative environment where each professional's expertise is valued [16]. Training programs should emphasize the importance of teamwork, communication, and the integration of services to provide comprehensive, patient-centered care. Collaborative care involves the integrated efforts of various healthcare professionals to provide comprehensive patient care.

Key professional roles

1. Primary care physicians (PCPs): PCPs often serve as the coordinators of care, ensuring that all aspects of a patient's health are addressed. They manage chronic conditions, provide preventive care, and facilitate referrals to specialists.

2. Nurses and nurse practitioners (NPs): Nurses and NPs play crucial roles in patient education, chronic disease management, and direct patient care. They often serve as the first point of contact for patients within the collaborative care team.

3. Mental health professionals: Psychologists, psychiatrists, and social workers provide necessary mental health support, integrating behavioral health into primary care. This integration is vital for treating conditions such as depression and anxiety that often co-occur with chronic physical health conditions.

4. Pharmacists: Pharmacists contribute by managing medication therapy, conducting medication reconciliation, and educating patients about their prescriptions. Their involvement helps optimize medication use and adherence.

5. Dietitians and nutritionists: These professionals offer dietary counseling and nutritional support, which is particularly important for patients with conditions such as diabetes, obesity, and cardiovascular diseases.

6. Physiotherapists: They assist in rehabilitation and management of physical conditions through exercises and therapeutic interventions, promoting mobility and physical function.

The insights above emphasize the critical roles that various healthcare professionals play in achieving collaborative care models. For example, a study that examined how individuals living with mental health issues access preventive care from their Physician to prevent complex health issues, integrated mental health services within primary care settings, showcases the collaborative efforts between primary care physicians and mental health professionals [10, 30]. This integration is shown to significantly improve patient outcomes, particularly in managing conditions like depression, adverse health conditions and incidence of falls among older adults. The pivotal role of pharmacists in managing polypharmacy among elderly patients is achieved from pharmacists' expertise in medication therapy management, which mitigate the risks of adverse drug interactions, thereby enhancing patient safety [31]. Nurse practitioners on the other hand, are essential in managing chronic diseases through patient education and direct care, which helps in controlling and reducing the impact of chronic conditions [23, 32]. The role of dietitians, underscores the importance of dietary counseling and nutritional support for patients with diabetes and cardiovascular diseases, contributing to better health management [22]. Lastly, the involvement of physiotherapists in rehabilitation, highlights their contribution to improving physical function and mobility through therapeutic interventions [13]. Collectively, these insights illustrate the importance of a multidisciplinary approach in providing comprehensive and effective patient care within the collaborative care model.

5.2 Addressing power imbalances and building trust

Developing strategies to address potential power imbalances and promote trust-based relationships between healthcare providers and population subgroups especially among underserved communities is critical. This can include engaging community members in the planning and decision-making processes, ensuring transparency in healthcare delivery, and creating feedback mechanisms that allow patients to voice their concerns and preferences. Building trust requires healthcare providers to demonstrate respect, empathy, and accountability consistently. By actively involving community members and addressing their specific needs and concerns, healthcare providers can foster stronger, more trusting relationships with the communities they serve. Power imbalances often arise from the hierarchical nature of healthcare professions, where certain roles, such as physicians, traditionally hold more authority compared to others, like nurses or social workers. This dynamic can hinder open communication and collaboration.

5.3 Strategies to address power imbalances

i. Interdisciplinary training: Providing joint training sessions for all team members can foster a better understanding of each role's contributions, promoting mutual respect.

ii. Shared decision-making: Encouraging shared decision-making processes where every team member's input is valued equally helps to balance power dynamics.

iii. Clear role definitions: Clearly defining roles and responsibilities ensures that each team member understands their scope of practice and respects others' expertise.

iv. Leadership development: Training leaders in collaborative care to recognize and mitigate power imbalances can create a more inclusive and equitable team environment.

5.4 Building trust

i. Open communication: Establishing regular, open communication channels helps build transparency and trust among team members.

ii. Team-building activities: Engaging in team-building activities can strengthen interpersonal relationships and trust within the team.

iii. Consistent meetings: Regular team meetings provide opportunities for discussing concerns, successes, and collaborative strategies, reinforcing trust and cohesion.

iv. Respect and empathy: Cultivating an environment where respect and empathy are prioritized helps build a culture of trust and support.

Addressing power imbalances and building trust are essential components of a successful collaborative care model. By implementing strategies that promote equality, open communication, and mutual respect, healthcare teams can enhance their collaboration, leading to better patient care and outcomes.

6. Contemporary and emerging measures

Assessing the impact of integrated care models on health equity requires the development and application of robust measures. These may include indicators of access, utilization, patient experiences, and clinical outcomes, disaggregated by race, ethnicity, socioeconomic status, and other relevant demographic characteristics [15]. Evaluating the efficacy and limitations of existing tools and measures for assessing the success of collaborative care in promoting health equity is also essential for identifying gaps and areas for improvement. Traditional measures often focus on clinical outcomes and service utilization but may overlook critical aspects such as patient satisfaction, cultural competency, and the broader social determinants of health. Emerging approaches, such as the use of artificial intelligence and machine learning, present opportunities to identify and mitigate biases in care delivery, but must be carefully designed and implemented to avoid perpetuating or amplifying disparities [32].

6.1 Existing tools and measures

Existing tools for assessing collaborative care often emphasize clinical outcomes and process measures [2, 4, 5]. These tools can provide valuable insights but may have limitations in capturing the full impact of care on underserved populations. For instance, they might not adequately account for social determinants of health or the unique challenges faced by specific demographic groups. To truly assess the efficacy of collaborative care models, it is crucial to use measures that reflect the lived experiences of patients and their overall well-being, beyond just clinical metrics, examples include measures where utilization focus on comprehensive care such as, ICOPE -for older populations, Community-based Care models for integrating local resources and health services and also Person-centered care frameworks for ensuring care plans are tailored to individual needs [8, 28–30] emphasizing the integration of health services to address physical, mental, and social health needs.

6.2 Emerging approaches and technologies

Emerging approaches and technologies present new opportunities for measuring the impact of collaborative care on social determinants of health within underserved communities. The use of artificial intelligence (AI) and machine learning can help identify patterns and predict outcomes, enabling more targeted interventions. However, these technologies must be carefully designed and implemented to avoid perpetuating or amplifying existing disparities. For example, algorithms used in AI must be trained on diverse datasets to ensure they do not reinforce biases present in the data. Additionally, real-time data analytics can provide ongoing feedback on the effectiveness of care interventions, allowing for continuous improvement and adaptation.

6.3 Evidence-base for contemporary and emerging measures

Analyzing the evidence base for contemporary and emerging measures in the context of collaborative care and health equity initiatives is vital for validating their effectiveness. Research has shown that integrating social determinants of health into assessment tools can lead to more comprehensive evaluations of health outcomes, other studies on the use of AI and machine learning in healthcare have demonstrated potential benefits in improving predictive accuracy and identifying at-risk populations, but they also highlight the importance of addressing ethical considerations and potential biases [13, 33]. Continuous research and validation are necessary to ensure these measures are reliable and equitable. By incorporating both contemporary and emerging measures, healthcare organizations can better assess the impact of integrated care models on health equity. These measures should not only focus on clinical outcomes but also consider patient experiences, access to care, and the broader social determinants of health. Utilizing advanced technologies like AI and machine learning, while ensuring ethical implementation, can enhance the ability to identify and address disparities in care delivery. Ultimately, robust and comprehensive measures are essential for advancing health equity and ensuring that integrated care models effectively serve all populations, particularly those who are underserved.

7. Research evidence in specific contexts

The effectiveness of integrated care models in reducing health disparities has been explored in various settings. For example, studies have examined the impact of integrated primary and specialist care on improving access and outcomes for marginalized populations with chronic conditions, such as diabetes and cardiovascular disease. Building on this evidence base, continued research in diverse contexts could be explored to reduce the cost of accessing healthcare through an interdisciplinary approach to meet the unique needs of underserved communities [33]. A few examples of practices that demonstrate why collaborative care is the best option to providing care to population subgroups.

7.1 Effectiveness of collaborative care models

Existing research has demonstrated the effectiveness of collaborative care models in addressing health disparities in specific underserved populations. For instance, rural communities often face unique challenges such as geographic isolation and limited healthcare resources. Studies have shown that integrated care models in these settings can significantly improve access to essential services, reduce travel time for patients, and enhance overall health outcomes [21]. Similarly, research focusing on racial and ethnic minorities has highlighted the benefits of culturally tailored collaborative care approaches in improving patient engagement, satisfaction, and clinical outcomes [6].

7.2 Promising practices and adaptations

Identifying promising practices and adaptations of collaborative care models within various community contexts including, disinvestment and interprofessional practice, is crucial for maximizing their impact. For example, among older adult populations, integrated care models that include components of geriatric care and social support have proven effective in managing chronic diseases and reducing hospital readmissions. In urban settings with high racial and ethnic diversity, employing community health workers and incorporating cultural competency training for providers have been shown to enhance the effectiveness of care delivery. These adaptations ensure that the care models are responsive to the specific needs and preferences of the populations they serve.

7.2.1 Disinvestment in health resources

The process of removing health resources from any current medical practices, procedures, technologies, or pharmaceuticals that are thought to provide little to no health benefit for their cost and are therefore inefficient uses of health resources is known as disinvestment [25]. According to the authors, both health providers and receivers bear the brunt of poorly managed healthcare systems. Also, a study by Elshaug and colleagues on policy makers' perspectives on disinvestments, the potential overutilization of less than effective clinical practices and the potential underutilization of effective clinical practices not only results in less-than-optimal care but also fragmented, inefficient, and unsustainable resource allocation [26]. Systematic policy approaches to disinvestment may improve efficiency as well as equity, quality, and safety of care, and perhaps even sustainability. It is therefore important that health policies that target these issues are tackled to allow for the advancement of the disinvestment agenda. This is a growing area of priority setting in health care that requires national and international perspectives, debate, and collaboration. Health policy can have a major impact on health and well-being. Healthy People 2030 focus on keeping people safe and healthy through laws and policies at the local, state, territorial, and federal level. This will ensure that people get timely, high-quality care services that they need [27].

7.2.2 Interprofessional practice (IPP)

Interprofessional practice (IPP) is a collaborative model in healthcare where multiple health professionals from different backgrounds work together with patients, families, and communities to provide care. The goal of IPP is to improve healthcare and reduce costs by combining the knowledge and skills of different providers to create a comprehensive, safe, and efficient system. Carey and colleagues suggest that there is evidence to support the relationship between interprofessional practice models (IPM) and health service equity for aging populations [34]. This fuels the need to improve collaborative practices between social care, public health care and health service providers to provide professional and ethical care to vulnerable populations and communities. Implications for practice relate to improving how interprofessional teams work with communities to achieve health care equity.

Case illustration

Equity can be described as being fair and impartial. In other words, putting things in place to make sure that people receive equal treatment regardless of the class that they belong to in society. As previously discussed, the goal of IPP is to improve healthcare and reduce costs by combining the knowledge and skills of different providers to create comprehensive, safe, efficient and ethical care to vulnerable populations and communities. A relatable example is the research findings from Alva, in a qualitative study that sought to understand First Year Experience FYE programs in the U.S. to understand students' experiences, explains the necessity for higher education to be "more intentional and intrusive in ensuring that underserved and underrepresented students attend academic workshops and employ the available resources to succeed" [35]. Several community colleges in three states were investigated on practices that promote equity in access to education. The study examined the ways in which FYE programs assist students who have historically encountered more challenges in obtaining and finishing higher education, and ways to overcome them. The findings suggest that, level of outreach efforts to reach underrepresented groups and economic issues were major hurdles to higher education access for this group [9]. Overall, both studies highlight the benefits of adopting an equity focus lens to increase low-income and underrepresented group access to education. The strategy includes, engaging, academic advisors from diverse cultural background, more retention and graduation specialists and institutions targeting support to students who have historically encountered more barriers to enrolling in and finishing their higher education. Likewise, healthcare systems that are equity focused in policy development recognizes the need to eliminate disparities in health outcomes among underserved and underrepresented populations.

7.2.3 Research findings synthesis

Synthesizing research findings from various studies helps to understand how collaborative care can contribute to long-term health equity and social justice for diverse underserved groups. Comprehensive analyses reveal that successful integrated care models share common elements such as strong community partnerships, patient-centered approaches, and flexibility to adapt to local contexts. These models not only improve immediate health outcomes but also build the capacity of healthcare systems to address social determinants of health and promote sustainable health equity. The evidence supports the notion that collaborative care can play a pivotal role in achieving social justice by ensuring that all individuals, regardless of their background or circumstances, have access to high-quality healthcare. In conclusion, continued research in diverse contexts is essential to further refine and adapt integrated care approaches to meet the unique needs of underserved communities. By analyzing existing research, identifying promising practices, and synthesizing findings, healthcare organizations and policymakers can develop and implement effective strategies to reduce health disparities and advance long-term health equity.

8. Policy-oriented interventions

Policy-level interventions can catalyze the adoption and sustainability of integrated care models that prioritize health equity. Aligning financial and non-financial incentives, such as payment reforms and value-based care initiatives, can motivate healthcare organizations to invest in the development and implementation of these models [11]. Policymakers and regulators must also ensure that the design and deployment of integrated care initiatives uphold principles of fairness and non-discrimination. In conclusion, integrated care models offer a promising approach to addressing health disparities in underserved populations. By enhancing access, addressing social determinants of health, and incorporating ethical considerations, these models have the potential to transform the healthcare landscape and advance health equity.

8.1 Evaluating current policies

To support the implementation and sustainability of collaborative care models in underserved communities, it is essential to evaluate current policies and propose evidence-based interventions. This involves analyzing existing healthcare policies to identify gaps and areas where enhancements can be made to better support integrated care. For example, policies that promote value-based care, where providers are reimbursed based on patient outcomes rather than services rendered, can incentivize the adoption of collaborative care models. Payment reforms that provide financial support for integrated care services, such as bundled payments or capitation, can further facilitate the sustainability of these models.

8.2 Identifying key stakeholders

Key stakeholders play a crucial role in promoting collaborative care for health equity. These stakeholders include policymakers, healthcare systems, community organizations, and patient advocates. Policymakers can create and enforce regulations that support integrated care, while healthcare systems can implement these models and adapt them to local needs. Community organizations are vital in engaging and educating the public, ensuring that care models are culturally appropriate and effectively address the community's needs. Patient advocates can provide valuable insights into patient experiences and help shape care models to be more patient-centered. Collaboration among these stakeholders is essential for the successful implementation of integrated care models.

8.3 Developing recommendations for policy changes

To empower stakeholders and advance collaborative care, developing recommendations for policy changes and resource allocation is critical. This includes advocating for increased funding for integrated care initiatives, ensuring that resources are directed towards underserved communities, and promoting policies that facilitate the training and retention of healthcare professionals in these areas. Additionally, policies should support the integration of social services with healthcare to address social determinants of health comprehensively. Recommendations may also include the creation of incentives for healthcare providers to participate in collaborative care models, such as tax benefits or grants.

Overall, integrated care models offer a promising approach to addressing health disparities in underserved populations. By enhancing access, addressing social determinants of health, and incorporating ethical considerations, these models have the potential to transform the healthcare landscape and advance health equity. Policy-level interventions that align incentives, involve key stakeholders, and promote fair and non-discriminatory practices are crucial for the successful adoption and sustainability of these models. Through strategic policy changes and resource allocation, stakeholders can be empowered to implement and maintain collaborative care models, ultimately achieving health equity for underserved populations.

9. Integrated and collaborative care impact

Integrated care practices offer substantial benefits to various population groups, particularly underserved, older adults, ethnic minorities and individuals who face complex health challenges. For elders, integrated care ensures coordinated management of multiple chronic conditions, reduces the risk of diseases, fragmented services and medical errors. By coordinating between primary, specialty, and geriatric care settings, access to care is enhanced while comprehensive health service is encouraged. Also, there's improved medication management, and interventions, leading to better overall health outcomes [29]. Additionally, as highlighted above and in the Appendix which with steps to achieving integrated care, patients' health providers can offer transportation assistance, social support, and community-based resources, to patients with mobility issues and those with difficulty accessing care, thus improving overall health outcomes [10]. Other underserved groups, such as rural communities and racial/ethnic minorities, can also benefit from improved access to care, reduced wait times, and culturally competent care that integrated models provide, ultimately fostering a more equitable healthcare system for all [19, 28, 36]. Collaborative care models provide a pragmatic strategy to deliver integrated mental health and medical care for persons with mental health care as mentioned earlier as demonstrated in the effectiveness of integrated care models for youth mental health, It addressed gaps in access to improve health outcomes by providing rapid access to services in a primary care setting, which was provided by a range of healthcare professionals, working together to manage patients' mental health needs, through effective utilization of resources. Thus, increasing access to mental health services, reduce stigma, provide holistic care and improved communication between providers and patients. Overall, this integration enabled young patients to receive treatment in a comfortable, easily accessible environment [37]. These models are also a cost-efficient strategy for primary care practices to improve outcomes for a range of mental health conditions across populations and settings.

Successful implementation of collaborative care models in routine care, however, require alignment of financial incentives to support system redesign investments, reimbursements for mental health providers, and other organizational and financial considerations [37]. Primary care has proven to ensure high levels of efficiency, effectiveness, equity, safety, timeliness and centrality of the patient, achieving better health outcomes and lower costs. The Chronic Care Model proposes a proactive approach in assisting the empowerment of patients and their community, contributing to improving the quality of care and health outcomes, as well as the reduction of inequalities [38]. Ultimately, integrated and collaborative care models hold significant promise in improving health equity across diverse populations by enhancing access, coordination, and the addressment of social determinants of health.

10. Conclusion

Integrated care models hold significant promise for advancing health equity and addressing the multifaceted health needs of underserved populations. The chapter address various levels of care, including programs to increase underrepresented populations' access to care, improve primary/secondary level care coordination using integrated health methods to improve population health outcomes. Some of the strategies include integrating clinical practice, primary, secondary and tertiary care in collaborative ways to improve practice. The examples provided in the Table and other Appendix show how well collaborative care models work, for example, the ICCT approach used to improve the mental health of young people, and how CHW programs work to close gaps between the healthcare system and the community to provide fair access to care. Although there are still obstacles to overcome before integrative care models can be successfully used to address disparities and complex health conditions, these examples show how they can improve health outcomes through community involvement and strong policy support. Healthcare access can be enhanced through reduced wait times, improved appointment availability, and transportation assistance, and effective partnerships among several sectors of service delivery using models that ensures marginalized communities receive comprehensive and patient-centered care. Ethical and professional considerations, such as cultural competency, informed consent, patient confidentiality, and interdisciplinary teamwork, are essential to the successful implementation of collaborative care. Furthermore, the development and application of robust measures, including emerging technologies like AI, are crucial for assessing the impact of these models on social determinants of health. Policy-level interventions also play a vital role in sustaining integrated care models. Aligning incentives, engaging key stakeholders, and promoting policy changes that support the integration of vital health services into primary care settings, and funding for integrated care models are essential. In addition, policies that promote infrastructure development, such as electronic health records to enable seamless communication between primary care and health providers and those that engage communities in the planning and implementation of integrated care models will ensure that the needs of various population subgroups are met. Despite the challenges of resource allocation in fostering collaboration among policymakers, healthcare systems, community organizations, patient advocates and institutions can create an inclusive and equitable healthcare system to enhance assess to care. There is need for continuous research, evidence synthesis, and strategic policy interventions that will ensure that integrated care models effectively reduce health disparities and promote long-term health equity - ultimately enabling all individuals to attain their full health potential. Integrated care practices offer substantial benefits to various population groups, particularly, for older adults who often face complex health challenges, this will ensure that care is coordinated in the management of multiple chronic conditions, as a result, mitigate the current fragmented care system and reduce medical errors.

In summary, reducing systemic healthcare disparities, particularly for underserved populations, can be achieved through transformative pathways such as achieving health equity through collaborative and integrative care models. The social determinants of health that underpin disparities are addressed by these models when primary, secondary, and tertiary care services are integrated. Effective programs like community health worker programs and collaborative care teams show promises for improving underprivileged communities' access to and quality of care. Geospatial analysis is one innovation that enhances healthcare planning and accessibility, highlighting the importance of data-driven strategies in resource allocation. But for progress to be sustained, strong legislative frameworks that encourage integration and give priority to cultural competency and strategies that involve communities are needed. All healthcare stakeholders should work together and make strategic investments to create an inclusive environment where everyone can achieve optimal health, regardless of socioeconomic status.

Conflict of interest

The authors declare no conflict of interest.

A. Appendix 1

Specific steps for implementing integrated care:

The following steps provide more insights into the implementation of integrated with the community health worker (CHW) led initiative:

1. Needs assessment

    Identify target population: Conduct a comprehensive needs assessment to identify the communities that would benefit most from CHW programs. This involves understanding the specific health challenges and social determinants affecting these populations.

    Engage stakeholders: Collaborate with community leaders, healthcare providers, and policymakers to design a CHW program that addresses identified needs and has community buy-in.

2. Program design

    Define roles and responsibilities: Clearly outline the roles and responsibilities of CHWs within the healthcare team. This includes determining the scope of practice, such as health education, patient navigation, and coordination of care.

Training and certification: Develop a robust training program for CHWs that covers essential skills, such as cultural competency, communication, and knowledge of healthcare systems.

3. Integration with healthcare systems

Collaborative approach: Foster collaboration between CHWs and healthcare providers by integrating CHWs into existing care teams. This requires establishing communication protocols and ensuring CHWs have access to necessary patient information.

Resource allocation: Secure funding and resources for the program, including salaries for CHWs and administrative support. Consider leveraging public and private funding sources to sustain the program.

Challenges to consider

1. Cultural barriers

CHWs often work within diverse communities with unique cultural practices and beliefs. It is crucial to ensure that CHWs are culturally competent and sensitive to these differences to build trust and effectively engage with the community.

2. Sustainability and funding

Securing long-term funding can be challenging. Programs must demonstrate their value to attract ongoing financial support. This requires developing a strong business case and communicating the program's impact on health outcomes and cost savings.

3. Integration and collaboration

Integrating CHWs into established healthcare systems can be challenging due to existing hierarchies and resistance to change. Overcoming these barriers requires strong leadership and clear communication about the benefits of CHW programs.

Metrics for evaluating success

1. Health outcomes

Measure improvements in specific health indicators, such as reduced hospital readmissions, improved management of chronic diseases, and increased rates of preventive care.

2. Patient satisfaction

Assess patient satisfaction with the care received, particularly regarding access to services and interactions with CHWs. Surveys and interviews can provide valuable feedback on program effectiveness.

3. Cost-effectiveness

Analyze the cost-effectiveness of the program by comparing healthcare utilization and costs before and after the implementation of the CHW program. Demonstrating a return on investment can support the case for sustaining and expanding the program.

B. Appendix 2

The summaries below reflect the content and themes presented in **Table 1**, highlighting the positive contributions, gaps, and factors influencing care, as well as focusing on different levels of care and relevant case studies.

Positive contributions to integrative care

Collaborative models: Articles highlight the success of integrated collaborative care teams, which improve service delivery, especially for mental health and substance use challenges among youth.

Community-based programs: Community health workers (CHWs) have been effectively integrated into primary care to address social determinants of health, leading to reduced healthcare utilization and costs.

Geospatial analysis: The use of geospatial analysis to map access to primary healthcare facilities has been pivotal in improving healthcare accessibility and planning.

Gaps in providing integrative care

Healthcare disparities: Significant gaps exist in healthcare access and outcomes, particularly among racial and ethnic minorities, as well as in rural and underserved communities.

Implementation challenges: There is a need for better frameworks to guide the implementation of integrated care models, particularly for complex conditions in older adults.

Factors influencing positive contributions

Community involvement: Successful integrative care models often involve strong community engagement and partnerships that empower local populations and improve health outcomes.

Policy and infrastructure: Policies that support interdisciplinary collaboration and the integration of healthcare services are crucial for advancing integrative care.

Case studies supporting collaborative health care youth mental health initiatives

Case studies on integrated collaborative care teams demonstrate their effectiveness in improving access and outcomes for youth with mental health and addiction challenge.

Community health worker programs

Case studies describe the impact of CHW programs in bridging gaps between communities and healthcare systems, promoting equitable access to care.

C. Appendix 3

Significant impact of community health initiatives and policy-making for integrated care

- Enhanced collaboration: The proposed generalizable approach encourages collaboration among various stakeholders, including county health systems, residency programs, public health departments, and local organizations. This collaboration is essential for addressing health disparities and improving health outcomes in underserved populations.

- Community health workers (promotors): The role of promotors is emphasized as a vital component in mobilizing community resources and addressing individual health needs. Their involvement can lead to better health outcomes by fostering community engagement and providing tailored support to patients.

- Focus on health equity: The integrative population health equity framework aims to advance health equity, particularly for Asian American communities. This framework can be applied to other underserved populations, highlighting the importance of culturally competent approaches in health interventions.

- Outcome measurement: The paper stresses the importance of population-based outcome metrics, such as reductions in hospitalizations and emergency department visits. By tracking these metrics, health organizations can assess the effectiveness of their initiatives and make data-driven decisions to improve service delivery.

- Addressing multi-level factors: The framework encourages understanding the multi- level contextual factors that influence health. This understanding can lead to more effective interventions that consider social determinants of health, ultimately improving community health outcomes.

- Sustainable health policies: The authors advocate for designing quality of care and payment policies that explicitly aim for health equity. This includes holding healthcare systems accountable through public monitoring and evaluation, which can lead to more sustainable health policies that benefit marginalized communities.

- Interdisciplinary approach: The paper highlights the need for an integrated, interdisciplinary approach to health care. By navigating funding sources and sustaining collaboration among various disciplines, health initiatives can be more effective in addressing complex health challenges.

In summary, the practical implications of emphasizing the importance of collaboration, community engagement, and a focus on health equity, can lead to improved health outcomes and more effective health policies for underserved populations.

DOI: http://dx.doi.org/10.5772/intechopen.1006809

Author details

Theresa Abah[1]* and Ifeyinwa Onwelumadu[2]

1 California State University, Sacramento, CA, United States

2 Southcentral Kentucky Community and Technical College, Bowling Green, Kentucky, United States

*Address all correspondence to: t.abah@csus.edu

References

[1] Ahmed A, Saqlain M, Tanveer M, Blebil AQ, Dujaili JA, Hasan SS. The impact of clinical pharmacist services on patient health outcomes in Pakistan: A systematic review. BMC Health Services Research [Internet]. 2021;**21**(1):1-14. Available from: https://link.springer.com/articles/10.1186/s12913-021-06897-0 [Accessed: July 18, 2024]

[2] Lawal O, Anyiam FE. Modelling geographic accessibility to primary health care facilities: Combining open data and geospatial analysis. Geo-spatial Information Science [Internet]. 2019;**22**(3):174-184. Available from: https://www.tandfonline.com/doi/abs/10.1080/10095020.2019.1645508 [Accessed: July 19, 2024]

[3] Aysola J, Bitton A, Zaslavsky AM, Ayanian JZ. Quality and equity of primary care with patient-centered medical homes: Results from a national survey. Medical Care [Internet]. 2013;**51**(1):68-77. Available from: https://journals.lww.com/lww-medicalcare/fulltext/2013/01000/quality_and_equity_of_primary_care_with.13.aspx [Accessed: July 18, 2024]

[4] Chin M, Drum M, Guillen M. Improving and sustaining diabetes care in community health centers with the health disparities collaboratives. Medical Care. 2007;**45**(12):1135-1143. Available from: https://journals.lww.com/lww-medicalcare/fulltext/2007/12000/Improving_and_Sustaining_Diabetes_Care_in.4.aspx [Accessed: July 14, 2024]

[5] Health Equity [Internet]. Available from: https://www.who.int/health-topics/health-equity [Accessed: July 20, 2024]

[6] Sherry M, Ghaffar A, Bishai D. Community platforms for public health interventions. In: Disease Control Priorities: Improving Health and Reducing Poverty. 3rd ed; 2017

[7] Chin DL, Bang H, Manickam RN, Romano PS. Rethinking thirty-day hospital readmissions: Shorter intervals might be better indicators of quality of care. Health Affairs. 2016;**35**(10):1867-1875

[8] Shahzad M, Upshur R, Donnelly P, Bharmal A, Wei X, Feng P, et al. A population-based approach to integrated healthcare delivery: A scoping review of clinical care and public health collaboration. BMC Public Health. 2019;**19**(1):708

[9] Cuellar MG, Gándara P. Promoting access and equity for underrepresented racial minorities? An examination of policies and practices in community college baccalaureate programs. Community College Review. 2021;**49**(1):52-75

[10] Henderson JL, Cheung A, Cleverley K, Chaim G, Moretti ME, De Oliveira C, et al. Integrated collaborative care teams to enhance service delivery to youth with mental health and substance use challenges: Protocol for a pragmatic randomised controlled trial. BMJ Open [Internet]. 2017;7(2):e014080. Available from: https://bmjopen.bmj.com/content/7/2/e014080 [Accessed: July 18, 2024]

[11] Gunderson JM, Wieland ML, Quirindongo-Cedeno O, Asiedu GB, Ridgeway JL, O'Brien MW, et al. Community health workers as an extension of care coordination in primary care: A community-based cosupervisory model. The Journal of Ambulatory Care Management. 2018;**41**(4):333-340

[12] Grossman E, Keegan T, Lessler A. Inside the health disparities collaboratives: A detailed exploration of quality improvement at community health centers. Medical Care. 2008. Available from: https://journals.lww.com/lww-medicalcare/fulltext/2008/05000/Does_the_Collaborative_Model_Improve_Care_for.7.aspx;**46**(5):489-496 [Accessed: July 14, 2024]

[13] Smith E, Lee A. COVID-19 and post-intensive care syndrome: Community-based care for ICU survivors. Home Health Care Management & Practice. 2021;**33**(2):117-124. DOI: 10.1177/1084822320974956

[14] Sadana R, Blas E, Budhwani S, Koller T, Paraje G. Healthy ageing: Raising awareness of inequalities, determinants, and what could be done to improve health equity. The Gerontologist. 2016; **56**(Suppl_2):S178-S193

[15] Fiscella K, Sanders MR. Racial and ethnic disparities in the quality of health care. Annual Review of Public Health [Internet]. 2016;**37**:375-394. Available from: https://www.annualreviews.org/content/journals/10.1146/annurev-publhealth-032315-021439 [Accessed: July 18, 2024]

[16] Andermann A. Taking action on the social determinants of health in clinical practice: A framework for health professionals. CMAJ [Internet]. 2016;**188** (17–18):E474-E483. Available from: https://www.cmaj.ca/content/188/17-18/E474 [Accessed: July 18, 2024]

[17] Castillo EG, Ijadi-Maghsoodi R, Shadravan S, Moore E, Mensah MO, Docherty M, et al. Community interventions to promote mental health and social equity. Current Psychiatry Reports. 2019;**21**(5):35

[18] Trinh-Shevrin C, Islam NS, Nadkarni S, Park R, Kwon SC. Defining an integrative approach for health promotion and disease prevention: A population health equity framework. Journal of Health Care for the Poor and Underserved. 2015;**26**(2):146-163

[19] Ornelas IJ. Cultural competency at the community level: A strategy for reducing racial and ethnic disparities. Cambridge Quarterly of Healthcare Ethics. 2008;**17**(2):185-194

[20] Moore AR, Lewis TH, Abah T, Celebi M, Amey FK. Examining participation disparities in cancer clinical trials. Oncology Nursing Forum [Internet]. 2023;**50**(1):79. Available from: https://openurl.ebsco.com/contentitem/doi:10.1188%2F23.ONF.79-89?sid=ebsco:plink:crawler&id=ebsco:doi:10.1188%2F23.ONF.79-89 [Accessed: July 20, 2024]

[21] Valaitis RK, Wong ST, MacDonald M, Martin-Misener R, O'Mara L, Meagher-Stewart D, et al. Addressing quadruple aims through primary care and public health collaboration: Ten Canadian case studies. BMC Public Health. 2020;**20**(1):507

[22] Chin MH. Advancing health equity in patient safety: A reckoning, challenge and opportunity [Internet]. BMJ Quality and Safety. 2021;**30**:356-361. Available from: http://qualitysafety.bmj.com/ [Accessed: July 18, 2024]

[23] De Carvalho IA, Epping-Jordan J, Pot AM, Kelley E, Toro N, Thiyagarajan JA, et al. Organizing integrated health-care services to meet older people's needs. Bulletin of the World Health Organization. 2017;**95**(11):756

[24] Bhardwaj A. Promise and provisos of artificial intelligence and machine learning in healthcare. Journal of Healthcare Leadership. 2022;**14**:113-118. Available from: https://www.

tandfonline.com/doi/abs/10.2147/JHL.S369498 [Accessed: July 20, 2024]

[25] Mitchell D, Bowles KA, O'Brien L, Bardoel A, Haines T. Health care staff responses to disinvestment—A systematic search and qualitative thematic synthesis. Health Care Management Review [Internet]. 2021;**46**(1):44-54. Available from: https://journals.lww.com/hcmrjournal/fulltext/2021/01000/health_care_staff_responses_to_disinvestment_a.6.aspx [Accessed: July 20, 2024]

[26] Elshaug AG, Hiller JE, Moss JR. Exploring policy-makers' perspectives on disinvestment from ineffective healthcare practices. International Journal of Technology Assessment in Health Care. 2008;**24**(1):1-9

[27] Health Care Access and Quality - Healthy People 2030. health.gov [Internet]. Available from: https://health.gov/healthypeople/objectives-and-data/browse-objectives/health-care-access-and-quality [Accessed: July 20, 2024]

[28] Leatt P, Pink GH, Guerriere M. Towards a Canadian model of integrated healthcare. Healthcare Papers. 2000;**1**(2):13-35

[29] Suragarn U, Hain D, Pfaff G. Approaches to enhance social connection in older adults: An integrative review of literature. Aging and Health Research [Internet]. 2021;**1**(3):100029. DOI: 10.1016/j.ahr.2021.100029

[30] Goodrich DE, Kilbourne AM, Nord KM, Bauer MS. Mental health collaborative care and its role in primary care settings. Current Psychiatry Reports [Internet]. 2013;**15**(8):1-12. Available from: https://link.springer.com/article/10.1007/s11920-013-0383-2 [Accessed: July 18, 2024]

[31] Midão L, Giardini A, Menditto E, Kardas P, Costa E. Polypharmacy prevalence among older adults based on the survey of health, ageing and retirement in Europe. Archives of Gerontology and Geriatrics. 2018;**78**:213-220

[32] Ferrer RL, Schlenker CG, Romero RL, Poursani R, Bazaldua O, Davidson D, et al. Advanced primary care in San Antonio: Linking practice and community strategies to improve health. Journal of the American Board of Family Medicine [Internet]. 2013;**26**(3):288-298. Available from: https://www.jabfm.org/content/26/3/288.short [Accessed: July 14, 2024]

[33] Abràmoff MD, Folk JC, Han DP, Walker JD, Williams DF, Russell SR, et al. Automated analysis of retinal images for detection of referable diabetic retinopathy. JAMA Ophthalmology [Internet]. 2013;**131**(3):351-357. Available from: https://jamanetwork.com/journals/jamaophthalmology/fullarticle/1668203 [Accessed: July 18, 2024]

[34] Carey MJ, Taylor M. The impact of interprofessional practice models on health service inequity: An integrative systematic review. Journal of Health Organization and Management. 2021;**35**(6):682-700

[35] Alva R. A Qualitative Study on the First-Year Experience of Underserved Students in the College of Business. Pomona: California State Polytechnic University; 2022. Available from: https://scholarworks.calstate.edu/concern/projects/pc289q867 [Accessed: July 20, 2024]

[36] Chin MH, King PT, Jones RG, Jones B, Ameratunga SN, Muramatsu N, et al. Lessons for achieving health equity comparing Aotearoa/New Zealand and the United States. Health Policy (New York). 2018;**122**(8):837-853

[37] Van Loenen T, Van Den Berg MJ, Heinemann S, Baker R, Faber MJ, Westert GP. Trends towards stronger primary care in three western European countries; 2006-2012. BMC Family Practice. 2016;**17**(1):59

[38] Thomson K, Bambra C, McNamara C, Huijts T, Todd A. The effects of public health policies on population health and health inequalities in European welfare states: Protocol for an umbrella review. Systematic Reviews [Internet]. 2016;**5** (1):57. DOI: 10.1186/s13643-016-0235-3

Chapter 8

Strategic Planning for Enhanced Healthcare Access in Macau: Focus on Medical Development and Resources

Chonin Cheang, Wengtong Chan and Suning Zhao

Abstract

This chapter provides a comprehensive analysis of strategic planning for enhanced healthcare access in Macau, focusing on medical development and resource optimization. It highlights the challenges and advancements in Macau's healthcare system, including restructuring, human resource development, and integration within the Guangdong-Hong Kong-Macao Greater Bay Area (GBA). Additionally, the chapter delves into the significant growth of the Traditional Chinese Medicine (TCM) industry, underpinned by robust legislative frameworks, academic achievements, and industrial collaborations. By examining Macau's healthcare policies, inter-regional cooperation, and innovative health solutions, this study aims to offer insights into creating a sustainable, high-quality healthcare system that addresses both current needs and future demands.

Keywords: Macau, healthcare, medical development, resources, planning

1. Introduction

Macau, a Special Administrative Region of China, has been undergoing significant developments and reforms in its healthcare system to improve healthcare access and services for its population. With a population of approximately 685,400, Macau faces the challenge of providing accessible and high-quality healthcare to its residents.

The system combines both public and private healthcare providers, including major public hospitals such as the Conde S. Januário Hospital, Kiang Wu Hospital, and The University Hospital (Macau University of Science and Technology Affilated Hospital), as well as numerous private clinics and healthcare facilities. This combination of public and private sectors aims to cater to the diverse healthcare needs of the population and enhance the overall healthcare infrastructure. To address the shortage of healthcare professionals, Macau is exploring recruitment and retention strategies. Efforts are being made to maximize the utilization of existing healthcare resources, reassess the manpower needs for service model transformation, and consider the involvement of healthcare professionals in non-nursing roles to alleviate the impact of nursing shortages. This strategic approach aims to ensure an adequate and skilled healthcare workforce to meet the growing demand for healthcare services [1].

Macau's integration with the Guangdong-Hong Kong-Macao Greater Bay Area (GBA) initiative presents opportunities for enhanced healthcare collaboration and development. The GBA includes cities such as Hong Kong and several other regions, creating a platform for knowledge exchange, resource sharing, and joint efforts to improve healthcare access and services [2]. Collaboration with healthcare providers in the GBA can help enhance the availability of specialized healthcare services and promote the overall development of the healthcare sector in Macau. In addition to general healthcare services, Macau is also focusing on the stable development of the traditional Chinese medicine (TCM) industry. The region has established research centers and academic institutions, such as the University of Macau and the Macau University of Science and Technology, to advance TCM research and education. Legislation, including the TCM Affairs and Chinese Medicine Registration Act, has been implemented to regulate and standardize TCM practices. These efforts aim to strengthen the TCM industry and promote its integration into the overall healthcare system in Macau.

Macau has been actively working toward enhancing healthcare access and services for its population. Through healthcare system restructuring, recruitment, and retention strategies, integration with the GBA initiative, and the development of the TCM industry, Macau aims to provide comprehensive and equitable healthcare services to its residents. These strategic initiatives are vital for meeting the healthcare needs of the population and ensuring the overall well-being of the community in Macau.

2. Healthcare system restructuring in Macau

Macau has implemented a mixed healthcare system, with both public and private healthcare institutions providing services. The healthcare system primarily serves the local population, which was approximately 685,400 as of the end of 2019. Major healthcare institutions in Macau include the Conde S. Januário Hospital, Kiang Wu Hospital, and The University Hospital, along with over 700 clinics. In 2019, the utilization of primary care services exceeded 4.1 million, including services provided by public healthcare facilities, private clinics, dental clinics, and TCM clinics. Health centers play a vital role in adult care, pediatric care, women's health, prenatal care, dental care, TCM, smoking cessation, and psychological counseling. Specialist outpatient services constitute the second-largest category of healthcare services in Macau, with over 1.89 million visits in 2019. Among these, 66% were handled by the Conde S. Januário Hospital, while the remaining cases were shared by private hospitals. Of the total cases, 16% of patients received government-subsidized services [3, 4].

The Health Bureau has set up vaccination points in schools, universities, and elderly homes to reduce transportation time for residents and enhance public health. In early 2020, when the COVID-19 pandemic emerged, the Macau government responded swiftly to ensure the safety of residents and healthcare workers. As a result, Macau has maintained a low infection rate [5, 6]. Timely and targeted measures have been implemented for disease prevention and control, diagnosis and treatment, and community education.

The healthcare system in Macau offers a variety of welfare programs. One key initiative is the Medical Subsidy Scheme, which has been in place since 2009. This scheme aims to share the economic benefits of social development with residents and alleviate their financial burdens. It promotes personal healthcare, leverages private healthcare institutions within community resources, and reduces pressure on public medical services. Additionally, it fosters a complementary relationship between public and private medical markets, thereby enhancing the overall quality of healthcare. In 2018, the scheme transitioned to an electronic medical voucher system, which facilitates the analysis, understanding, and oversight of voucher usage [3, 7].

Medical subsidies are available for residents who present their Macau Resident Identity Card. They are exempted from primary healthcare fees at health centers and receive a 30% discount on healthcare fees at the Conde S. Januário Hospital for specialist care. Free medical services are provided at the Conde S. Januário Hospital for specific groups, including pregnant women, civil servants and their dependents, teachers, children aged 10 and below, primary and secondary school students, and individuals aged 65 and above [3, 8].

The financial resources for public healthcare services in Macau primarily come from taxes, with the healthcare budget allocated by the Cultural Affairs Bureau accounting for approximately 70% of healthcare expenditure. The remaining costs are covered by patient payments, which account for around 30% of healthcare expenditure. Private insurance companies contribute only a small proportion. Healthcare expenditure in Macau has been increasing in recent years, from MOP 6391.4 million in 2015 to MOP 8395.2 million in 2019. The proportion of healthcare expenditure to government spending has remained high during this period. The Health Bureau's actual revenue was approximately MOP 7.99 billion, with a year-on-year increase of 9.9%. Total expenditure was approximately MOP 7.69 billion, with a year-on-year increase of 6.9%. The investment expenditure for the Health Bureau's development plan in 2019 was approximately MOP 1.5 billion, with an execution rate of 84.1%. Compared to neighboring regions or economies, individual healthcare expenditure in Macau has remained relatively low. In 2019, healthcare expenditure accounted for 2.5% of GDP, indicating a continuous increase in healthcare spending. This is attributed to the Macau Health Bureau's efforts to improve healthcare services, establish an electronic health record exchange system, and strengthen disease surveillance, reporting, drug reserves, and vaccination programs [3, 8, 9].

In addition, the Health Bureau in Macau has established an online organ donation registration page. As of the end of 2019, over 4100 individuals have registered as organ donors [3]. The Health Bureau has also strengthened cooperation with non-profit and private medical institutions, purchasing approximately 845,000 medical services from 13 non-profit medical institutions. These services include Western and Chinese medicine outpatient services, periodontal treatment, dental sealants for schoolchildren, home care, cervical cancer screening, psychological therapy, and other referral services. Furthermore, seven non-profit medical institutions receive funding for health promotion and training activities. The government's Public Health Laboratory receives approximately 117,000 samples annually, with a 14% year-on-year increase. The total number of tests exceeds 341,000, with an 8% year-on-year increase. Virus testing accounts for the majority of samples, representing 64.8% of the total and 76.8% of the total number of tests [3, 7].

Macau has implemented a mixed healthcare system that provides comprehensive healthcare services to its residents. The system includes both public and private healthcare institutions, ensuring access to high-quality medical services. The government has implemented various policies and measures to provide medical subsidies and welfare, reducing the financial burden on residents. Macau's healthcare resources have been invested in and developed with financial support, aiming to improve the quality and level of healthcare services. Collaboration with neighboring regions, such as Hong Kong, and participation in international initiatives, including the World Health Organization, contribute to the enhancement of disease prevention and control, as well as the overall healthcare standards in Macau. The implementation of smart healthcare initiatives, including electronic systems and data analysis platforms, further promotes healthcare information technology. Overall, Macau's healthcare system is designed to provide comprehensive healthcare services for its residents [3, 4].

3. Human resource development

3.1 A comparative analysis of Macau and other comparable regions in medical human resource

To analyze the medical human resource of Macau, a comparative analysis of Macau and other countries is needed to show the advantages and challenges of medical human resource in Macau. Here, Hong Kong, Malaysia, and Singapore were chosen as comparable areas as they are relatively small countries or areas in Southeast Asia. **Table 1** shows the vital statistics of the four jurisdictions, including Macau, Hong Kong, Malaysia, and Singapore. In general, Macau has a younger population (median age: 38.0) with a relatively higher percentage of population aged 65 or above (13.3%) and a medium annual population growth (1.27%).

Table 2 shows the health system data, including service provision and health expenditure. All the jurisdictions have a mixed health system, i.e., a public-private provider and financing system. The funding mechanism is mainly through general taxation, except in Singapore having an additional medical savings account [17]. Macau has a lower healthcare spending per capita (US$ 1818) and total health expenditure as per GDP (2.6%) [17]. However, Macau's public health expenditure as a percentage of total health expenditure is the highest of the four mixed health system jurisdictions (74.1%) [18].

Table 3 shows the manpower statistics. In 2018, Macau shows the highest ratio of doctors (2.6) but the second lowest of nurses (3.7) per thousand population [18].

In Hong Kong, the ratio of nurses to patients at public hospitals stands at one nurse to 12 patients, taking into consideration the high occupancy rate and

Indicators	HK [10, 11]	Malaysia [12]	Singapore [13, 14]	Macau [15]
No. of Population (in '000)	7674	32,700	5640	673
Median age	45.6	30.3	42.1	38.0
No. of population aged ≥65 (%)	20	6.3	3.8	13.3
Annual population growth rate (%)	0.8	1.2	2.2	1.1
Infant mortality rate (per 1000 registered live births)	1.6	7.3	2.2	1.9
Life expectancy at birth (Years)				
Male	80.7	72.7	80.7	80.9
Female	86.8	77.4	85.2	86.7

Table 1.
The general statistics between four regions (2022).

Indicators	HK [16]	Malaysia [17]	Singapore [17]	Macau [15]
Health system	Mixed health system	Mixed health system	Mixed health system	Mixed health system
Funding mechanism	Tax-based funding	Tax-based funding	Tax-based medical savings account	Tax-based funding
Health spending per capita ($US)	2195	262	2462	1818
% share of inpatient services provision (public vs. private)	90:10	73:27	80:20	36:64
% share of outpatient services provision (public vs. private)	30:70	60:40	20:80	20:80
Total health expenditure as % of GDP	5.7	3.8	4.5	2.6
Public health expenditure as % of total health expenditure	48.9	51.4	54.5	74.1
Out-of-pocket expenditure as % of total health expenditure	34.0	37.6	31.2	NA

Table 2.
Health system data between four regions (2017).

Indicators	HK	Malaysia	Singapore	Macau
No. of doctors per 1000 population	1.93	1.61	2.20	2.60
No. of nurses per 1000 population	7.13	3.08	7.20	3.70

Table 3.
The manpower statistics between four regions.

additional patients in the ward, way below the international standard of one to six [19]. Currently, doctors' ratio is 1.93, while nurses' ratio is 7.13 per 1000 population (**Table 3**). It is expected additional 1669 nurse and 1007 doctor headcounts are needed by 2030 to catch up with population growth [20].

In Malaysia, the 2014 nurse ratio is 3.08 per 1000 population (**Table 3**) [21]. 2016 doctors' ratio was 1.61. By 2020, it is expected to need 130,000 nurses in all specialties [22], where an additional 37,319 nurses are needed to meet the International Council of Nurses (ICN) recommended ratio of 5.00 per 1000 population) [23]. Meanwhile, an additional 4354 doctors are needed by 2020 [11].

In Singapore, the current nurse ratio per 1000 populations is 7.2 (**Table 3**) [24], and that of doctors for 2016 is 2.2, which is below the ratio of the USA (2.6) [25] and Macau. With the projected aged population in Singapore reaching 610,000 and 960,000 by 2020 and 2030, it is anticipated they would need an additional 30,000 healthcare workers by 2020 to cope with the aging population. From MOH, extra 5504 doctors are needed by 2027 [26].

Manpower shortage is a universal problem. Although the causes are complex and varied among different countries, the root of this healthcare crisis can simply be summarized as "the decreased supply cannot meet the increased demand" [27]. This chapter begins with the specific factors underpinning the increased demand, followed by factors contributing to the decreased supply of manpower. Those challenges can be divided into four areas [18]:

- Increasing demand from demographic shift: in Asia, one-third of the population in HK will be aged 65 by 2064. In Singapore, the elderly population is projected to be 610,000 and 960,000 by 2020 and 2030, which is 32.6% and 109% more when compared to 2015 [28], whereas in Malaysia, the total elderly population will be 3.4 million by 2020. Such changes in population imply changes in the healthcare utilization pattern as people present more complex needs that may require a heightened level of medical care and demand for healthcare resources. The hospital bed use requirement of those aged 65 or above is about nine times more than that of younger people, and the average stay for the elderly is 9.7 days, as compared to 5.3 days for non-elderly patients [20].

- Poor workforce planning: In Malaysia, there was an oversupply of student nurses from 2005 to 2010, producing 10,000 nurse graduates per year. The overproduction compromised the quality of student nurses. Consequently, criticisms of poor service quality and nurse image were reported. In order to uphold the quality, MNB announced new regulations in 2010, increasing nursing entry requirements from three to five credits. Moreover, a drop in National Higher Education Fund Corporation (PTPTN) loans for students from RM 60,000 to 38,000 forced many colleges offering nursing courses to close, resulting in reduced nurse supply. Currently, the yearly production is less than 3000 nurses [22].

- Low morale: In HK, with the booming private healthcare industries, demand for nurses in the private sector increases. Private healthcare service providers offer a higher salary package in order to increase market competitiveness. The public service is under challenge due to the manpower shortage. The outflow was worsening the morale of nurses who are working under high workload pressure in HA. The nurse outflow from the public sector was 2.1% and 4.7% in 2005 and 2009, respectively. A record-high outflow rate of 5.7% was reported of public doctors in 2018 [29]. In Singapore, in 2010, public doctors' attrition rate was 10% due to the big income gap of 1.7–10 times in the private sector. In Malaysia, many students put nursing careers at a lower priority than other disciplines [30] because of unfavorable employment conditions, including low salaries, poor working conditions, and a lack of professional recognition from a low education entry requirement. In addition, there is a disparity in the distribution of doctors. With 5–10 times higher income in private practice, the 4427 specialists (56%) staying in the public sector are serving 80% of the population, while the 3412 specialists (44%) take care of the remaining 20% in 2016. Moreover, the retention rate of doctors in rural areas of Sabah and Sarawak is low (40%). Most doctors found themselves practicing in urbanized West Malaysia, e.g., Wilayah Persekutuan, Kular Lumpur, Selangor, Penang, Perak, and Johor [31].

- Medical tourism: A distinctive feature of Southeast Asia is its engagement in medical tourism. Singapore and Malaysia have emerged as major destinations of international patient flows. In 2015, 300,000 and 400,000 patients traveled to Malaysia and Singapore, respectively, for treatments [32]. Singapore and Malaysia import health workers to meet domestic demand and to provide services to international patients. This situation has resulted in the so-called brain drain of highly specialized staff from public to private hospitals. Meanwhile, Malaysia slips into a nation of training and exporting nurses to neighboring countries, which further results in the migration of Malaysian Building a High Quality and Sustainable Healthcare System Delivery in Macau Page 56 healthcare manpower, especially to Singapore, the Middle East, the UK, the US, and Australia. With respect to the movement of health workers for medical tourism, banning nurse migration is widely recognized as neither possible nor ethical. One route to addressing this challenge has therefore been to establish codes of practice for the international recruitment of health personnel [33]. It is voluntary in nature and achieved through bilateral agreements covering agreed numbers of migrants. However, the diversity of the ASEAN region, including differences between countries in the quality of education and training, licensing requirements, language, and cultural dimensions of medical practice, makes implementation of these agreements very challenging [32].

To tackle manpower shortages, the interventions used in those regions can be organized into five priority areas, as shown in **Table 4**, which provides experiences to Macau for medical human resource planning.

3.2 The planning of human resource development in Macau

3.2.1 Medical manpower

Macau has a higher doctor-to-population ratio compared to Hong Kong, Singapore, and the United Kingdom. However, the doctor-to-population ratio varies widely and would depend on the model of care, whether it is primary care-led or heavily hospital care-based. The number of specialists required for each individual specialty is also important, and a detailed breakdown of the required specialists for

Themes	Sub-themes
(a) Macroeconomics and health sector funding	—
(b) Workforce planning and policy	• Increase training places and facilities. • Professional development, e.g., expanding new roles for nurses • Creating more assisting roles
(c) Positive practice environments	• Staff engagement • Strengthen the supportive infrastructure • Occupational Health & Safety Promotion
(d) Retention and recruitment	• Increase salary/allowance • Encouraging overseas recruitment • Education programs to attract non-nursing disciplines to join the nursing profession • Encourage lapsed nurses/doctors to return to practice • Addressing gaps between education and services, e.g., mentoring
(e) Leadership	• Independent nursing organization establishment • Leadership program • Improving image of nursing, e.g., image campaign

Table 4.
Interventions to tackle manpower shortages categorized by five priority areas.

the different specialty is beyond the scope of this consultancy, and is more appropriately done by the Academy of Medicine in collaboration with all the different specialties. There are certain specialties and subspecialties that would need to be developed in the near future after the formation of the Macau Academy of Medicine, such as psychiatry, geriatrics, and occupational medicine. With the setting up of the local medical school, be it a private one, there will come a time when Macau would need to consider whether doctors returning from overseas would need to be assessed formally through a Licensing Examination or continue with the status quo. Macau should review the need to develop medical specialties currently not available in Macau or in the public system in the interest of Macau citizens (e.g., occupational medicine) and consider sending people to other countries for the training if appropriate [18].

The demand-based projection model predicts that Macau will need to train up more doctors in the longer term to meet increasing service demands and the opening of the new hospital. Since the increase in doctors required for the private clinics and the two small private hospitals will be subject to economic cycles, the projection for this part would not be too reliable. The increase in doctors needed for public and KWH, University Hospital together, in 2021 will be 125, and in 2026 it will be 302 (compared with the 2016 baseline and did not include doctors in administration offices) [18].

The Macau government should work together with the Macau Academy of Medicine to determine the specialist requirement in due course and the development of new specialties and subspecialties. With the local medical school coming into shape, the long-term policy and practical arrangement for doctors returning from overseas would need to be reviewed [18].

3.2.2 Nursing and other healthcare professionals

To address the nursing shortage in particular in the private and community sector and the expected increase in demand in all sectors with the aging population and to prepare for the opening of the new hospital in 2023, Macau Health Bureau will have to take early and prompt action, including [18]:

- Recruitment strategies: It includes increasing nursing school intake and overseas recruitment. From our projection, increasing the intake of nursing school by 25% in 2019 could keep the supply–demand in balance until 2026. Measures to attract school leavers to pursue nursing as a life-long career are needed.

- Retention strategies: It includes decreasing resignation rates and extending retirement age. An enhancement in the career structure, pathway, and recognition is required. Professionalism can be motivational with an educational approach for learning and improvement.

- Maximizing nursing resources: Nursing manpower planning should consider maximizing nursing roles and responsibilities according to the population healthcare needs. For example, nursing specialization could be considered in particular for those specific areas in need, such as geriatric or community nurses, in view of aging population, which would reduce nursing demand from avoidable hospitalization. Ways to reduce non-nursing duties to give nurses more time to deal with nursing work would help to retain more nurses in the health system, as described in paragraphs 8.77 and 8.79. Fractional appointments for nurses who have retired or are not in active employment could be considered.

While nurses can serve different roles in healthcare, other healthcare professionals could be recruited to perform some borderline nursing duties currently undertaken by nurses. Apart from the nurse assistants, occupational therapists and medical social workers could take up the roles of case managers and assist in navigating the services for patients. Macau should explore into expanding their roles in due course and relieve the work of nurses [18].

Macau should explore into recruitment and retention strategies; maximize nursing resources to increase the nursing workforce for the whole of Macau; reassess manpower needs on service model changes; and consider how other healthcare professionals with the appropriate skill mix could take up some non-nursing roles, such as case managers, to relieve the impact of the shortage of nurses [18].

4. Integrated healthcare in the GBA

4.1 Background

GBA is a region in southern China, encompassing nine cities and two special administrative regions. As the most expansive and densely populated urban area in southern China, the GBA has a population of over 86 million and spans an area of 56,000 km^2 [34, 35]. The healthcare industry and facilities have undergone significant expansion in parallel with the advancement of socioeconomic development [36]. As a result of its status as a Special Administrative Region of China, Macau has benefited considerably from the GBA initiative, particularly in the area of healthcare. One of the most evident strengths of the MSAR healthcare system is the relatively equitable access to healthcare services that it provides to all its residents. The emphasis on primary care is a significant strength of the Macau healthcare system. However, the MSAR has been observed to have a relatively limited range of specialist options available to its residents. In 2019, the cost of transfers to other jurisdictions for treatment not available in the MSAR was MOP 218 million [15]. Residents in Macau, particularly those afflicted with challenging, complex, and rare diseases, are frequently transferred to Hong Kong, Guangzhou, and Shenzhen in pursuit of more advanced medical care. In view of the growing demand for healthcare, the escalating costs of medical care, the expansion of specialized medical services, and the risk of infectious diseases, Macau has planned to adopt the strategy of integrating healthcare in the GBA to ensure the provision of a higher standard of healthcare for its residents.

4.2 The integration and collaboration trend in the GBA

The healthcare sector in the GBA is experiencing significant integration and collaboration, driven by various initiatives and policies designed to create a more unified and efficient healthcare system. In these years, the primary initiatives mainly include joint hospitals and clinics, telemedicine and remote consultations, joint research initiatives, cross-border health insurance, and emergency response coordination. Among these initiatives, the establishment of joint hospitals and clinics has made huge progress. Healthcare providers in the GBA are forming joint ventures to establish hospitals and clinics that serve patients from across the region. One of the most notable examples is the University of Hong Kong-Shenzhen Hospital (HKU-SZH), which is a joint project between the University of Hong Kong and the Shenzhen Municipal Government.

HKU-SZH was opened in 2012, which is the first "Hong Kong-style public hospital" in Shenzhen, as described in the newspaper [37]. It has a total floor area of 367,000 square meters and a total land area of 192,000 square meters, with 2000 beds currently in operation and a total capital cost of approximately four billion Yuan [6]. In less than a decade, it has been awarded Australian Council on Healthcare Standards accreditation and was granted the status of a 'Grade 3A' hospital, which is the highest ranking of the national hospital accreditation system of mainland China. Located on the border of Shenzhen and Hong Kong, the hospital was expected to integrate the best Western model of healthcare delivery with the best Chinese model. It has been working assiduously on this integration and has made notable progress.

As a vital part in GBA integration, HKU-SZH is implementing a multitude of initiatives that are currently underway [38]:

- HKSAR Elderly Healthcare Voucher (EHCV): The EHCV, which was launched in 2015, has the objective of facilitating access to healthcare services at HKU-SZH for Hong Kong elders who are residents of Shenzhen, the Pearl River Delta area, and Hong Kong. The voucher enables eligible Hong Kong elders to pay for outpatient services provided by HKU-SZH. Since its inception, HKU-SZH has documented over 45,000 instances of EHCV patient episodes or outpatient attendances [2].

- Pilot Scheme for Supporting HA Patients in GBA: In order to facilitate the development, residence, and integration of Hong Kong citizens in the mainland, the Government of the Hong Kong Special Administrative Region initiated the Pilot Scheme for Supporting Patients of the Hospital Authority in the GBA (Pilot Scheme) on May 10, 2023. In light of the experience gained from the Special Support Scheme during the course of the 2019 coronavirus pandemic, patients with scheduled follow-up appointments at either Specialist Outpatient Clinics or General Outpatient Clinics of the Hospital Authority are able to receive subsidized consultations at HKU-SZH.

- Shenzhen Hospital Accreditation Research Center: The Shenzhen Hospital Accreditation Research Center was officially registered and established in December 2020 with the objective of developing a hospital evaluation and accreditation system that adheres to international standards, implementing internationalized hospital accreditation methods, and advancing the internationalization of hospital accreditation in China.

- Shenzhen-Hong Kong Medical Specialties Training Center: In July 2019, the SZ-HK Medical Specialist Training Center was inaugurated at HKU-SZH. The hospital has introduced an international medical education and training system, drawing on the talent training experience of Hong Kong and foreign countries. This system is designed to meet international standards and to be recognized in China. The center is structured into two principal committees: the Governance Committee and the Executive Committee. In accordance with the national standardized residency training system, the "3 + 4" specialist training framework has been established, comprising three years of national residency training and four years of specialist training in Shenzhen and Hong Kong. The center intends to provide training in nine specialties and has developed preliminary training programs.

- Drugs and Equipment Introduced from HK/Macau: HKU-SZH is the pioneering medical institution for the pilot introduction of drugs and medical devices in urgent clinical use that have been listed in Hong Kong and Macau but have not been approved for registration by the National Medical Products Administration (NMPA). These drugs and devices cannot be replaced by registered varieties on the Chinese mainland, as outlined in the Work Plan for Supervision, Innovation, and Development of Drugs and Medical Devices in GBA (2020) [39]. As of December 2021, thirteen pharmaceuticals and three medical devices had been approved under the aforementioned measure. These drugs and medical devices have been introduced into clinical practice, thereby conferring tangible benefits on patients.

Moreover, HKU-SZH functions as a gateway to facilitate convenient healthcare access for residents of Hong Kong and Shenzhen. Subsequently, the University of Hong Kong-Shenzhen Hospital-Hospital Authority clinics (HKU-SZH-HA) were also established in 2021. During the five-month trial period, a total of 11,000 inquiries and 10,938 patient episodes or clinic attendances were recorded [2]. Although the clinics were constrained in terms of the range of services they offered, it was of paramount importance to demonstrate that integrated medical care is an effective and sustainable model.

The integration of healthcare in GBA is exemplified by the response to the pandemic caused by the SARS-CoV-2 virus. In the context of the fifth wave of the SARS-CoV-2 pandemic in Hong Kong, the deployment of healthcare personnel from mainland China commenced in mid-March 2022. A total of 391 medical personnel, primarily from Guangdong Province, were deployed to the community treatment facility at Asia World-Expo. They worked in close collaboration with their Hong Kong counterparts to combat the pandemic [40]. The positive experiences and encounters of medical workers on both sides during the COVID-19 pandemic have led to the belief that mutual learning, concern, assistance, and cooperation, between the two different medical systems are achievable and will be helpful in providing quality healthcare in the GBA and beyond.

4.3 Macau union hospital: A collaboration of Macau and Peking union medical college hospital

The Islands Healthcare Complex—Macau Medical Center of Peking Union Medical College Hospital (Macau Union Hospital) represents a further instance of integration in the GBA area, with the HKU-SZH model providing a point of reference. It is a large-scale, comprehensive public medical institution established by the Government of the Macau Special Administrative Region (Macau SAR) and managed by the Macau SAR and Peking Union Medical College Hospital (PUMCH). The hospital commenced operations on a trial basis in December 2023, with official commencement scheduled for September 2024. The facility occupies an area of approximately 76,000 square meters, with a total built-up area of approximately 430,000 square meters. The complex is designed to accommodate 800 beds and 26 operating rooms. It will include the Macau Hospital, the Logistics and Support Building, the Residential Building for Staff, the Administration and Multi-Services Building, and the Central Laboratory Building [41].

Macau Union Hospital is a jointly operated institution with the objective of fulfilling the need for specialist and high-quality healthcare for Macau residents. Additionally, it is tasked with addressing the challenges posed by an aging population and the potential for infectious disease outbreaks. PUMCH, one of the most esteemed medical institutions in China, boasts a wealth of expertise in hospital administration and operations, accumulated over centuries. The experiences and resources they possess can be leveraged to provide advanced healthcare services in Macau, as exemplified by HKU-SZH, which has enhanced healthcare services in Shenzhen through the efforts of the University of Hong Kong. The new hospital has 700 beds, which represents an increase of approximately 30% in the total number of hospital beds in Macau (2149 in 2020) [41]. Besides, Macau Union Hospital introduces advanced medical facilities to Macau, such as AI adaptive intelligence radiotherapy systems and all-round linear accelerators integrating new irradiation technology for cancer patients. These advancements enable the hospital to meet the sophisticated healthcare needs of Macau residents.

Furthermore, Macau Union Hospital has the potential to serve as a catalyst for the growth of medical tourism. In addition to offering superior healthcare services, the facility is equipped to treat patients with complex and rare diseases from other GBA cities, thereby facilitating the integration of healthcare in GBA at a higher level.

5. Steady progress in the TCM industry

Recent advancements in Macau's pharmaceutical sector, particularly in TCM, highlight a strategic alignment between educational achievements, legislative developments, and industrial collaboration. The University of Macau and the Macau University of Science and Technology, ranking 193rd and between 251–300th, respectively, in the 2024 Times Higher Education (THE) rankings [42], underscore the territory's commitment to research and academic excellence. These institutions are pivotal research hubs, significantly contributing to the pharmaceutical sector, especially in R&D in Chinese medicine. On the legislative front, the enactment of the "Law on TCM Affairs and Registration of Proprietary Chinese Medicines" along with its "Implementation Rules" on January 1, 2022, marks a significant milestone [43]. These legal frameworks have been instrumental in regulating and standardizing practices within the TCM industry, ensuring they meet local and international standards. The establishment of the Macau Pharmaceutical Administration Bureau in the same year further reinforced this regulatory infrastructure, enhancing the systematization of drug regulations and promoting the internationalization of Macau's pharmaceutical products [44].

In terms of infrastructure and international collaboration, Macau has established itself as a significant player. The WHO Collaborating Centre for Traditional Medicine (Macau) serves as a focal point for TCM on the global stage, facilitating international cooperation. Additionally, the State Key Laboratory of Quality Research in Chinese Medicine, a joint initiative between the University of Macau and the Macau University of Science and Technology, plays a crucial role in elevating research standards and ensuring products meet international quality benchmarks [45]. The Guangdong-Macau Traditional Chinese Medicine Technology Industrial Park symbolizes regional collaboration, acting as a hub for innovation and production. It bridges traditional methods with modern technology and practices, supporting the scale-up of production that adheres to Good Manufacturing Practice (GMP) standards applicable in both mainland China and the European Union. This compliance is crucial for Macau's vision to export TCM products to international markets, ensuring they meet rigorous safety and efficacy standards. Furthermore, Macau's strategy to become a hub for pilot production and R&D transformation in TCM is successful, attracting over 200 enterprises related to TCM, health products, medical devices, and medical services. This influx of enterprises is a direct result of the supportive ecosystem that includes robust academic research, stringent regulatory frameworks, and state-of-the-art industrial facilities [45–47].

These concerted efforts have positioned Macau as an international player in the pharmaceutical and TCM industries, paving the way for future developments and collaborations that could further propel Macau onto the global stage.

5.1 Development of TCM academic disciplines and talent cultivation

Both the University of Macau and the Macau University of Science and Technology have established disciplines related to the TCM industry. These institutions actively collaborate with mainland China and international universities to co-develop academic programs in medicine and pharmaceutical sciences, facilitating the joint cultivation of talents well-versed in both theoretical knowledge and practical applications. These universities leverage state-of-the-art facilities such as national key laboratories to provide students with excellent learning and research opportunities [45]. Collaborations with renowned educational and research institutions enhance the quality of education and research capabilities, preparing students to contribute effectively to the TCM industry. A significant initiative in talent development is the role played by the Guangdong-Macau Traditional Chinese Medicine Technology Industrial Park. This park serves as an international hub for young TCM practitioners, offering specialized training programs in TCM culture and techniques. These programs nurture young professionals from Macau and abroad, fostering a new generation of specialists equipped with both traditional and modern medicinal knowledge. Furthermore, through partnerships with the mainland China Drug Administration and the WHO Collaborating Centre for Traditional Medicine, Macau enhances the training of regulatory professionals and establishes a platform for international exchange and cooperation. These efforts integrate Macau's TCM industry with global practices and standards [45, 46]. Additionally, the Macau government's talent attraction scheme plays a vital role in driving the development of the local TCM industry. By recruiting top global talents and leveraging their expertise, experiences, and networks, Macau enhances its local capabilities and positions itself as a leader in the global TCM market. This strategy enriches the local talent pool and ensures the continuous advancement and internationalization of Macau's TCM sector [48].

5.2 Improving the TCM management system

The Macau government has rigorously implemented legal and regulatory frameworks to enhance the governance of TCM. The enactment of the "Traditional Chinese Medicine and Proprietary Chinese Medicine Registration Act" and accompanying regulations has established a robust system for the approval, registration, and management of TCM [43]. This includes supporting local Chinese medicine manufacturers in adopting GMP standards, thereby standardizing TCM activities and fortifying the registration system for proprietary Chinese medicines to improve quality control and safety oversight. An innovative evaluation and approval system that blends TCM theories, empirical human usage, and clinical trials has been developed. This system permits the incorporation of real-world data and other safety information to replace certain pharmacological, toxicological studies, or early-stage clinical trials, ensuring the quality and safety of both innovative and improved pharmaceuticals. In addition to pharmaceuticals, a regulatory framework for medical devices and cosmetics has been implemented to enhance their quality and safety, safeguarding public health [44, 45]. This framework aligns with Macau's strategic vision for medical tourism, supporting the development, research, and production of these products and driving industry growth. Capitalizing on national policies and Macau's geographical advantages, the government is attracting high-quality enterprises to develop medical devices, cosmetics, and associated industries locally. It promotes a collaborative model that integrates TCM, medical devices, and cosmetics, aiming to nurture emerging sectors and diversify the overall health industry [44–46].

To optimize the business environment for the TCM and broader health industries, the government has established ongoing communication channels with enterprises, offering comprehensive, one-stop lifecycle services [45]. These proactive initiatives help businesses understand and navigate the development landscape, providing tailored support and assistance. Enterprises benefit from pre-registration consultation services for proprietary Chinese medicines, which demystify the registration process and reduce R&D risks, thereby accelerating market entry. Moreover, the government continuously improves service commitments related to drug registration and licensing, enhances approval processes, develops intelligent drug regulatory systems, and optimizes electronic services. These improvements create a conducive business environment, increase administrative efficiency, and bolster investor confidence in the industry [46].

5.3 Innovation and research cooperation

Macau has strategically positioned itself as a global leader in TCM through a comprehensive ecosystem that fosters innovation through close collaboration among academia, industry, and research institutions. This ecosystem is robustly supported by the partnership between the University of Macau and the Macau University of Science and Technology at the State Key Laboratory of Quality Research in Chinese Medicine. Here, pioneering research is conducted to advance methodologies ensuring quality and safety in TCM, meeting both national and international standards. The State Key Laboratory drives forward exploratory and innovative projects that bridge traditional medicine with modern technological applications, transforming theoretical research into market-ready TCM products. This enhances the laboratory's capabilities and significantly boosts Macau's reputation within the international TCM community, keeping the region at the forefront of TCM technology and practices.

Supplementing these research initiatives, the Macau Institute for Applied Research in Medicine and Health plays a crucial role in translating scientific breakthroughs into practical, commercial applications. This institute integrates technological innovation with talent development, efficiently coordinating with local and regional networks to fast-track the technology transfer process, ensuring swift transition of innovations from the lab to the market. In parallel, the Macau Center for R&D in Chinese Medicine cultivates critical partnerships with leading pharmaceutical enterprises from mainland China, focusing on the development of classical TCM prescriptions and establishing a comprehensive "variety-quality-brand" system. This system ensures high-quality TCM products and fosters a strong brand reputation for Macau's TCM industry internationally.

The integration of the Guangdong-Macau Traditional Chinese Medicine Technology Industrial Park into this framework provides a state-of-the-art platform for scaling up and commercializing TCM products. Meeting GMP standards of both mainland China and the European Union, the park offers facilities optimized for both pilot production and large-scale manufacturing of TCM, supporting services from contracted research and development to quality enhancement and registration filings [45]. The Macau Society for Health Economics also plays a vital role in this integrated ecosystem by optimizing economic policies within the healthcare sector. This society conducts research that supports decision-making processes related to healthcare financing and economic sustainability in TCM, ensuring that economic considerations align with scientific advancements and market dynamics [48].

Furthermore, Macau's strategic initiatives encompass the integration of TCM with health and wellness tourism. Facilities like the Macau Concord Hospital not only enhance Macau's appeal as a destination for medical tourism but also demonstrate the region's unique capability to blend TCM with comprehensive health management services. Through these interconnected efforts, Macau not only confirms its status as a pioneering center for TCM but also establishes a robust framework for the sustainable development of the health and wellness sectors. This aligns with its vision of becoming a global destination for tourism and healthcare, highlighting the effective transformation of scientific research into technological and commercial achievements in the TCM sector.

5.4 Regional cooperation in the TCM industry

In recent years, Macau has strategically leveraged its geographic and cultural position to become a central node in the network of TCM within the GBA. This collaboration is guided by the comprehensive framework set forth in the "Guangdong-Hong Kong-Macau Greater Bay Area Traditional Chinese Medicine Development Plan (2020-2025)." This plan aims to enhance the regional TCM industry by fostering a collaborative environment that overcomes legal, regulatory, and systemic barriers, facilitating a smoother flow of medicinal products, professionals, and healthcare practices across borders [49]. Macau's role in this initiative is multifaceted, focusing on integrating resources, research, and regulatory frameworks. One key strategy has been to encourage the establishment of cross-border medical facilities and partnerships. These facilities not only serve as bases for exchanging medical expertise and training but also act as frontiers for the clinical application of TCM innovations developed within Macau's research institutions.

6. Future directions and sustainability

Looking ahead, Macau's healthcare system faces several key opportunities and challenges. Sustainability will hinge on continuous innovation in healthcare services and the integration of advanced technologies like AI and telemedicine. The development of human resources, particularly through increased training capacities and enhanced recruitment strategies, remains crucial. Furthermore, strengthening collaborations within the GBA will be vital for sharing resources and expertise, especially in handling complex health challenges and pandemics.

The TCM industry's future will likely focus on expanding international markets, requiring adherence to global standards and increased research capabilities. Macau must also continue to develop policies that support the seamless integration of TCM into mainstream healthcare, promoting its acceptance and use both locally and globally.

Environmental sustainability should also be a priority, with the healthcare sector adopting greener practices and contributing to the broader environmental goals of the region. This includes minimizing waste, promoting sustainable procurement practices, and ensuring that new healthcare facilities are built to eco-friendly standards.

7. Conclusion

Macau's strategic approach to healthcare reform and development has set a foundation for addressing both immediate and long-term health challenges. Through a mix of policy innovation, strategic collaborations, and resource optimization, Macau has enhanced its healthcare access and quality. The ongoing development of the TCM industry, coupled with the integration efforts in the Greater Bay Area, positions Macau to continue its trajectory toward becoming a leader in healthcare innovation and sustainability. Ultimately, the region's commitment to improving healthcare outcomes and fostering a sustainable future reflects its dedication to ensuring the well-being of its residents in an ever-evolving global health landscape.

Conflict of interest

The authors declare no conflict of interest.

Appendixes and nomenclature

TCM	Traditional Chinese Medicine
GBA	Guangdong-Hong Kong-Macao Greater Bay Area

Author details

Chonin Cheang*, Wengtong Chan and Suning Zhao
Macau Society for Health Economics, Macau SAR, China

*Address all correspondence to: zhengjunxianalex@gmail.com

References

[1] Macao Magazine. Macao's Union Hospital: A Milestone for the City's Health System. 2024. Available from: https://macaomagazine.net/macao-union-hospital-macau/ [Accessed: 21 July 2024]

[2] Pai PMC, Fan JKM, Wong WCW, Deng XF, Xu XP, Lo CM. Promoting integrated healthcare for Hong Kong and Macau residents in the Greater Bay Area during the COVID-19 pandemic. Hong Kong Medical Journal. 2023;**29**(3): 268-272. DOI: 10.12809/hkmj2210229

[3] Health Bureau of the Government of the Macao Special Administrative Region. Health-Related Activities Coordination of Public and Private Organizations [Internet]. Available from: https://www.cdqq.gov.mo/en/home-coming/living/health-social-welfare/ [Accessed: 21 July 2024]

[4] How Macau's Health Care System was Primed to Beat the Pandemic, Despite only Opening a Medical School Months Ago [Internet]. Available from: https://www.scmp.com/magazines/post-magazine/long-reads/article/3081268/how-macaus-health-care-system-was-primed-beat [Accessed: 21 July 2024]

[5] Ung COL, Hu Y, Hu H, Bian Y. Investigating the intention to receive the COVID-19 vaccination in Macao: Implications for vaccination strategies. BMC Infectious Diseases. 2022;**22**(1):218. DOI: 10.1186/s12879-022-07191-y

[6] McCartney G, Pinto J. Macao's COVID-19 responses: From virus elimination success to vaccination rollout challenges. The Lancet Regional Health – Western Pacific. 2021;**11**:100169. DOI: 10.1016/j.lanwpc.2021.100169

[7] Macau News. Digital Health Vouchers Reduce Medical Subsidy Scheme Violations Macau: Macau News. 2022. Available from: https://macaonews.org/news/community/digital-health-vouchers-reduce-medical-subsidy-scheme-violations/ [Accessed: 21 July 2024]

[8] Telecommunications Bureau of Macao. Macau Telecommunications Report 2024 [Internet]. Macau: Telecommunications Bureau of Macao; 2024. Available from: https://www.tdm.com.mo/en/news-detail/957460 Accessed: 21 July 2024

[9] Hong Kong-Macau-Medical Equipment|Privacy Shield. n.d.. Available from: https://www.privacyshield.gov/ps/article?id=Hong-Kong-Macau-medical-equipment [Accessed: 21 July 2024]

[10] Census and Statistics Department Hong Kong Special Administrative Region. Hong Kong Population Projections 2015-2064 [Internet]. 2015. Available from: http://www.statistics.gov.hk/pub/B1120015062015XXXXB0100.pdf

[11] Department of Health. Health Statistics [Internet]. 2022. Available from: https://www.dh.gov.hk/english/statistics/statistics_hs/statistics_hs.html

[12] Department of Statistics Malaysia Official Portal. MyDemography [Internet]. 2024. Available from: https://www.dosm.gov.my/portal-main/online-services?data=6

[13] Department of Statistics Singapore. Population Trends Dashboard [Internet]. 2024. Available from: https://www.singstat.gov.sg/find-data/search-by-theme/population/population-and-

population-structure/visualising-data/population-trends-dashboard

[14] Department of Statistics Singapore. Death and Life Expectancy [Internet]. 2024. Available from: https://www.singstat.gov.sg/find-data/search-by-theme/population/death-and-life-expectancy/latest-data

[15] Government of Macao Special Administrative Region Statistics and Census Service. Statistical Data [Internet]. 2024. Available from: https://www.dsec.gov.mo/en-US/?NodeGuid=ba1a4eab-213a-48a3-8fbb-962d15dc6f87

[16] Department of Health. Health Facts of Hong Kong 2017 Edition [Internet]. 2017. Available from: https://www.dh.gov.hk/english/statistics/statistics_hs/files/2017.pdf

[17] World Bank Group. DataBank [Internet]. 2024. Available from: https://databank.worldbank.org/

[18] Macao Health Bureau. Building a High Quality and Sustainable healthcare System Delivery in Macao [Internet]. 2019. Available from: https://www.ssm.gov.mo/docs/16808/16808_895b148a230247a89383a7fa57d634ed_000.pdf [Accessed: 15 July 2024]

[19] Keung F. Urgent Need to Increase Supply of Nurses in HK [Internet]. 2016. Available from: http://www.chinadailyasia.com/opinion/2016-06/27/content_1545413 3.html

[20] Food and Health Bureau of HKSAR. Government Strategic Review on Manpower Planning and Professional Development [Internet]. 2017. Available from: https://www.legco.gov.hk/yr19-20/english/panels/hs/papers/hs_e.htm

[21] Ministry of Health Malaysia. Health Facts [Internet]. 2015. Available from: https://myhdw.moh.gov.my/public/pub?p_p_id=110_INSTANCE_QUU93ji8Vrjk&p_p_lifecycle=0&p_p_state=normal&p_p_mode=view&p_p_col_id=column-1&p_p_col_count=1&_110_INSTANCE_QUU93ji8Vrjk_struts_action=%2Fdocument_library_display%2Fview_file_entry&_110_INSTANCE_QUU93ji8Vrjk_fileEntryId=150212

[22] Pillay S. Will Malaysia Faces a Nurse Shortage by 2020? The Strait Times Online [Internet]. 2017. Available from: https://www.nst.com.my/news/2017/01/201014/will-malaysia-face-sh ortage-nurses-2020

[23] Goh JM. Malaysia to Face a Nursing Shortage by 2020. MIMS Today [Internet]. 2017. Available from: https://today.mims.com/malaysia-to-face-a-nursing-shortage-by-202 0

[24] Singapore department of Statistics. 2017 Singapore in Figure [Internet]. 2017. Available from: https://www.singstat.gov.sg/-/media/files/publications/reference/sif20 17.pdf

[25] OECD Publishing. A System of Health Accounts: 2011 Edition [Internet]. 2017. Available from: https://www.oecd.org/en/publications/a-system-of-health-accounts-2011_9789264270985-en.html

[26] Yang MA. Student Learning Blog of NUS-ISS-Analytics and Intelligent Systems Practice Group, Healthcare Manpower Shortage in Next 10 Years [Internet]. 2017. Available from: https://analyticsandintelligentsystems.wordpress.com/2017/08/06/he althcare-manpower-shortage-in-next-10-years/

[27] Oulton JA. The global nursing shortage: An overview of issues and actions. Policy, Politics & Nursing Practice. 2006;7(Suppl. 3):34S-39S. DOI: 10.1177/1527154406293968

[28] Singapore Ministry of Health. Singapore Healthcare Manpower Plan 2020: Care for the Nation, Transforming Tomorrow's Healthcare [Internet]. 2019. Available from: https://www.moh.gov.sg/docs/librariesprovider5/pressroom/highlights/2020-healthcare-manpower-plan.pdf

[29] South China Morning Post. Record-High Doctors' Turnover Rate of 5.7% in Hong Kong Public Hospitals Worsens Manpower Shortage Issues [Internet]. 2018. Available from: www.scmp.com/news/hong-kong/health-environment/article/2127176/record-high-doctors-turnover-rate-57-cent-hong

[30] Barnett T, Namasivayam P, Narudin DA. A critical review of the nursing shortage in Malaysia. International Nursing Review. 2010;**57**(1):32-39. DOI: 10.1111/j.1466-7657.2009.00784.x

[31] Rahim RA, Mwanri L. Health workforce crisis: Recruitment and retention of skilled health Workers in the Public Health Sector in Malaysia. Asia Pacific Journal of Public Administration. 2012;**34**(2):157-170. DOI: 10.1080/23276665.2012.10779392

[32] Kanchanachitra C, Lindelow M, Johnston T, et al. Human resources for health in Southeast Asia: Shortages, distributional challenges, and international trade in health services. Lancet. 2011;**377**(9767):769-781. DOI: 10.1016/S0140-6736(10)62035-1

[33] World Health Organisation. Models and Tools for Health Workforce Planning and Projections. Geneva, Switzerland: World Health Organisation; 2010. Available from: https://iris.who.int/bitstream/handle/10665/44263/9789241599016_eng.pdf?sequence=1&isAllowed=y

[34] Xie J, Ren C, Li X, Chung LCH. Investigate the urban growth and urban-rural gradients based on local climate zones (1999-2019) in the Greater Bay Area, China. Remote Sensing Applications: Society and Environment. 2022;**25**:100669. DOI: 10.1016/j.rsase.2021.100669

[35] Zhang Y, Chen Z, Tang B, Sun H. Analysis of Spatio-temporal characteristics of urban economic resilience and influencing factors in Guangdong-Hong Kong-Macao Greater Bay Area. Frontiers in Public Health. 2022;**10**:922096. DOI: 10.3389/fpubh.2022.922096

[36] Fu G, Li J, Geng P, et al. A study on COVID-19 prevention force of typical cities in the Guangdong-Hong Kong-Macau Greater Bay area based on the medical perspective. China Biotechnology. 2022;**41**(12):125-140. DOI: 10.13523/j.cb.2108040

[37] Wikipedia. University of Hong Kong-Shenzhen Hospital [Internet]. 2024. Available from: https://en.wikipedia.org/wiki/University_of_Hong_Kong%E2%80%93Shenzhen_Hospital

[38] The University of Hong Kong. Shenzhen Hospital. About Us [Internet]. 2024. Available from: http://www.hku-szh.org/xgdxszyy/yygk/xwzx/index_14.html

[39] Greater Bay Area. Access of Drugs and Medical Devices [Internet]. 2022. Available from: https://www.bayarea.gov.hk/gbais/en/development/medical-co-operation/allowing-designated-healthcare-institutions-in-the-greater-bay-area-to-use-hong-kong-registered-drugs-and-medical-devices/

[40] Li Y. HKSAR Chief Executive Sees Off Mainland Medical Workers Supporting Pandemic Fight. Chinanews.

com [Internet]. 2022. Available from: http://www.ecns.cn/news/2022-05-06/detail-ihayamfc5315102.shtml. [Accessed: 5 June 2022]

[41] The Islands Healthcare Complex. Macao Medical Center of Peking Union Medical College Hospital. About Us [Internet]. 2024. Available from: https://www.cmm-pumch.gov.mo/en/about-us-en/introduction-en

[42] Times Higher Education. World University Rankings 2024 [Internet]. 2024. Available from: https://www.timeshighereducation.com/world-university-rankings/2024/world-ranking [Accessed: 15 July 2024]

[43] Macau S.A.R. Government. Lei da Actividade Farmacêutica no Âmbito da Medicina Tradicional Chinesa e do Registo de Medicamentos Tradicionais Chineses [Internet]. 2021. Available from: https://bo.io.gov.mo/bo/i/2021/30/lei11.asp#11 [Accessed: 15 July 2024]

[44] Macau S.A.R. Government. Instituto Para a Supervisão e Administração Farmacêutica [Internet]. 2021. Available from: https://www.io.gov.mo/pt/legis/rec/14640?md5__1263=n4%2Bx0DyDnG5QqhDBuYoYGQr40KjRxwqY5x&alichlgref=https%3A%2F%2Fwww.io.gov.mo%2Fcn%2Flegis%2Frec%2F14640%3Fmd5__1263%3Deq**Ax0DBD9**DgiYRDBktDyDmOja70QQkK4D%26alichlgref%3Dhttps%253A%252F%252Fwww.google.com%252F [Accessed: 15 July 2024]

[45] Macau S.A.R. Government. Moderate Economic Diversification Development Plan of the Macau Special Administrative Region (2024-2028) [Internet]. 2023. Available from: https://www.dsepdr.gov.mo/uploads/attachment/2023-10/e-book_C.pdf [Accessed: 15 July 2024]

[46] State Key Laboratory of Quality Research in Chinese Medicine (University of Macau). The Innovative Achievements of Traditional Chinese Medicine are Gradually Implemented, and the Results of Government Support are Beginning to Show [Internet]. 2024. Available from: https://sklqrcm.um.edu.mo/%e4%b8%ad%e8%97%a5%e5%89%b5%e6%96%b0%e6%88%90%e6%9e%9c%e6%97%a5%e6%bc%b8%e8%90%bd%e5%9c%b0-%e6%94%bf%e5%ba%9c%e6%94%af%e6%8c%81%e6%88%90%e6%95%88%e5%88%9d%e9%a1%af/ [Accessed: 15 July 2024]

[47] The Talent Development Committee of Macau S.A.R Government. Introduction and Legislation of the Talent Recruitment System [Interent]. 2023. Available from: https://www.cdqq.gov.mo/en/talent-recruitment-system/ [Accessed: 15 July 2024]

[48] Macau S.A.R. Government. Society of Health Economics [Internet]. 2024. Available from: https://www.io.gov.mo/cn/entities/priv/rec/11886?md5__1263=n4%2Bx9DBD0DyiitNi%3DKDsf3hxmhiDuAlZ62i3D&alichlgref=https%3A%2F%2Fwww.google.com%2F [Accessed: 15 July 2024]

[49] China Administration of Traditional Chinese Medicine. Guangdong-Hong Kong-Macau Greater Bay Area Traditional Chinese Medicine Development Plan (2020-2025) Press Release and Work Deployment Meeting [Internet]. 2020. Available from: http://www.natcm.gov.cn/guohesi/gongzuodongtai/2020-11-11/18139.html [Accessed: 15 July 2024]